ECG Interpretation

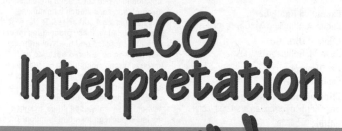

an Incredibly Easy!®

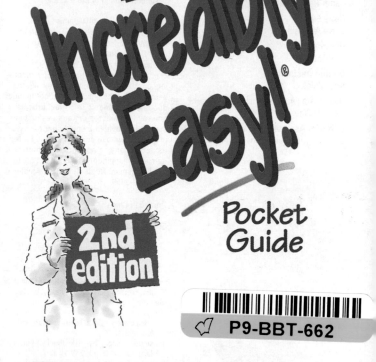

Pocket Guide

2nd edition

Wolters Kluwer | Lippincott Williams & Wilkins
Health

Philadelphia • Baltimore • New York • London
Buenos Aires • Hong Kong • Sydney • Tokyo

P9-BBT-662

Staff

Executive Publisher
Judith A. Schilling McCann, RN, MSN

Clinical Director
Joan M. Robinson, RN, MSN

Art Director
Elaine Kasmer

Clinical Project Manager
Jennifer Meyering, RN, BSN, MS, CCRN

Editor
Diane Labus

Clinical Editors
Dorothy P. Terry, RN
Janet Rader Clark, RN, BSN

Copy Editor
Jerry Altobelli

Illustrator
Bot Roda

Design Assistant
Kate Zulak

Associate Manufacturing Manager
Beth J. Welsh

Editorial Assistants
Karen J. Kirk, Jeri O'Shea, Linda K. Ruhf

Printed in China

ECGIEPG2E—010709

Library of Congress Cataloging-in-Publication Data
ECG interpretation : an incredibly easy! pocket guide.—2nd ed.
      p. ; cm.
   Includes bibliographical references and index.
ISBN 978-1-60547-251-5
   1. Electrocardiography—Handbooks, manuals, etc. I. Lippincott Williams & Wilkins.
   [DNLM: 1. Electrocardiography—nursing—Handbooks. 2. Arrhythmias, Cardiac—nursing—Handbooks. WG 39 E17 2010]
RC683.5.E5.E2534 2010
616.1'207547—dc22   2009014230

RRS0904

Contents

Contributors and consultants

Diane M. Allen, RN, MSN, ANP-BC, CLS
Nurse Practitioner
Womack Army Medical Center
Fort Bragg, N.C.

Karen Crisfulla, MSN, CCRN
Clinical Nurse Specialist—
  Electrophysiology
Hospital of the University
  of Pennsylvania
Philadelphia

Leslie L. Davis, RN, MSN, ANP-C
Predoctoral Teaching Fellow
University of North Carolina
Chapel Hill

Louise Diehl-Oplinger, RN, MSN,
  CCRN, ACNS-BC, NP-C
Nurse Practitioner—Practice Owner
Lehigh Valley Wellness Center
Phillipsburg, N.J.

Mary Lou Fisher, RN, MSN, CRNP, CCRN
Health and Nutrition Advisor
Samaritan's Purse
Boone, N.C.

Deborah A. Hanes, RN, MSN, CNS, NP
Clinical Nurse Specialist
Ohio State University Medical Center—
  The James Cancer Hospital
Columbus

Johnette Kay, RN, BSN
Instructor, Practical Nursing Program
Our Lady of the Lake College
Health Careers Institute
Baton Rouge, La.

Merita Konstantacos, RN, MSN
Staff Nurse CVSICU/CVSD
Aultman Hospital
Canton, Ohio

Roger Scott, BN, NP, EMT-P, ENC(C)
Nurse Practitioner
1 Field Ambulance Edmonton
  (Alberta) Clinic

Allison J. Terry, RN, PhD, MSN
Director, Center for Nursing
Alabama Board of Nursing
Montgomery

Wynona Wiggins, RN, MSN, CCRN
Assistant Professor of Nursing
Arkansas State University
State University

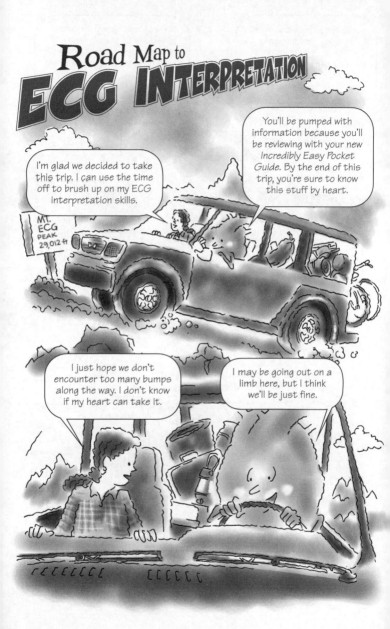

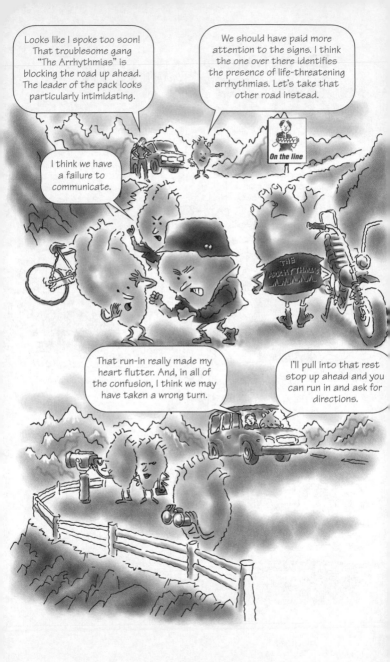

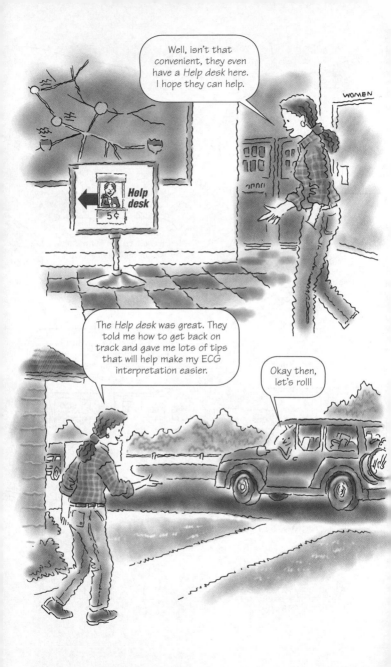

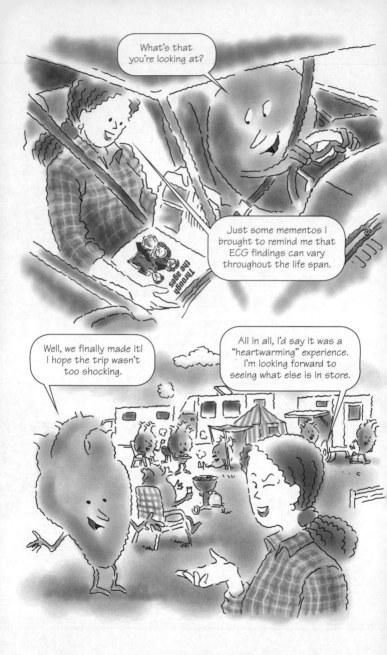

Basic electrocardiography

1

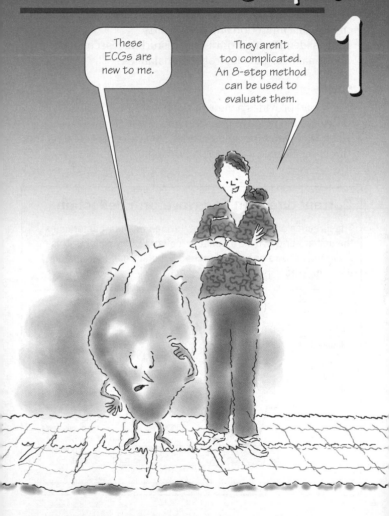

Electrocardiogram review

- Records the heart's electrical activity as waveforms that depict depolarization (contraction) and repolarization (relaxation)
- Is used to diagnose and monitor certain disorders, such as myocardial infarction and pericarditis
- Allows identification of rhythm disturbances, conduction abnormalities, and electrolyte imbalances

Leads

- Each lead provides a view of the heart's electrical activity between one positive pole and one negative pole.
- Each lead generates characteristic waveforms based on the direction electrical current is flowing.

Current direction and waveform deflection

The direction of electrical current through the heart determines the upward or downward deflection of an ECG waveform. This illustration shows possible directions of electrical current and their corresponding waveform deflections.

As current travels toward the negative pole, the waveform deflects mostly downward.

When current flows perpendicular to the lead, the waveform may be small or deflect in both directions (biphasic).

As current travels toward the positive pole, the waveform deflects mostly upward.

Planes

- Each plane is a cross section of the heart that provides a different view of the heart's electrical activity.
- The six limb leads are viewed from the frontal plane.
- The six precordial leads are viewed from the horizontal plane.

12-lead ECG

- Records information on 12 different views of the heart using a series of electrodes placed on the patient's limbs and chest
- Six limb leads (I, II, III, aV_R, aV_L, aV_F)
  – Provide information about the frontal plane of the heart
  – May be bipolar and thus require a negative and positive electrode for monitoring (leads I, II, and III)
  – May be unipolar and thus need only a positive electrode (augmented leads aV_R, aV_L, and aV_F)
- Six precordial leads (V_1, V_2, V_3, V_4, V_5, V_6)
  – Provide information about the horizontal plane of the heart
  – Are unipolar (need only a positive electrode)
  – Allow calculation of the negative pole of the lead (in the center of the heart) by the ECG monitor

Single-lead or dual-lead ECG

- Monitor up to two different leads
- Display heart rate
- Commonly monitored leads
  – I, II, and III
  – MCL_1 and MCL_6 (modified chest leads, similar to unipolar leads V_1 and V_6 of the 12-lead ECG, which are also used in dual-lead monitoring)

Help desk

Dual-lead monitoring

Monitoring in two leads provides a more complete picture than monitoring in one. Therefore, if it's available, dual-lead monitoring should be used to detect ectopy or aberrant rhythms.

With simultaneous dual monitoring, the first lead — usually designated as the primary lead (lead II) — is reviewed for arrhythmias. The second lead (lead V_1) helps detect ectopic beats or aberrant rhythms. Leads II and V_1 are the leads most commonly monitored simultaneously.

Lead II

Lead V_1

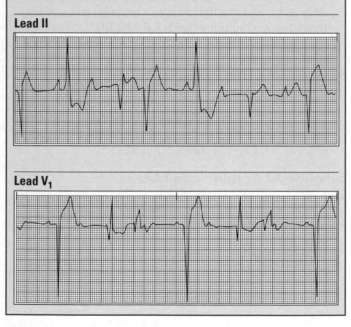

ECG monitoring systems

- May be hardwire or telemetry based on the patient's clinical status
- Hardwire monitoring
  - Permits continuous observation of one or more patients from more than one area of the unit
  - Connects electrodes directly to cardiac monitor
  - Limits mobility (patient is tethered to a monitor)
  - Provides a continuous cardiac rate and rhythm display
  - Transmits the ECG tracing to a console at the nurses' station
  - Has alarms
  - Has attachments that can track pulse oximetry, blood pressure, hemodynamic status, and other values
- Telemetry monitoring
  - Allows mobility (patient carries a small, battery-powered transmitter that sends electrical signals to another location for display on a monitor)
  - Useful for detecting arrhythmias during rest, sleep, exercise, and stressful situations
  - Monitors only heart rate and rhythm

ECG monitoring systems may work by hardwire or telemetry.

Electrodes and electrode placement

- Electrodes are adhesive pads with conductive gel that are attached to the patient's skin.
- Leadwires attach (clip or snap on) to the electrodes.
- Electrode placement is different for each lead.
- Different leads provide different views of the heart.
- A three- or five-electrode (or leadwire) system may be used for cardiac monitoring.

Standard limb leads

- Lead I
  - Positive electrode on the left arm
  - Negative electrode on the right arm
  - Positive deflection
  - Helpful in monitoring atrial rhythms
- Lead II
  - Positive electrode on the left leg
  - Negative electrode on the right arm
  - Positive, high-voltage deflection resulting in tall P, R, and T waves
  - Useful for identifying P waves, detecting sinus node and atrial arrhythmias, and monitoring the inferior wall of the left ventricle
- Lead III
  - Positive electrode on the left leg
  - Negative electrode on the left arm
  - Positive deflection
  - Useful for monitoring atrial rhythms and the inferior wall of the left ventricle

(Text continues on page 9.)

Einthoven's triangle

The axes of the three bipolar limb leads (I, II, and III) form a shape known as *Einthoven's triangle*. Because the electrodes for these leads are about equidistant from the heart, the triangle is equilateral.

The axis of lead I extends from shoulder to shoulder, with the right-arm lead being the negative electrode and the left-arm lead being the positive electrode. The axis of lead II runs from the negative right-arm lead electrode to the positive left-leg lead electrode. The axis of lead III extends from the negative left arm lead electrode to the positive left leg lead electrode.

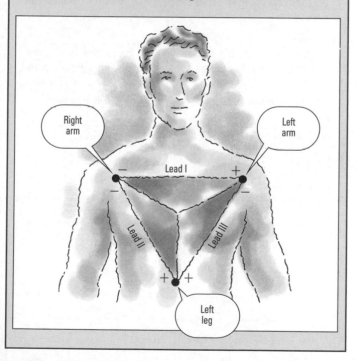

Leadwire systems

These illustrations show the correct electrode positions for some of the leads you'll use most often—the five-leadwire, three-leadwire, and telemetry systems. In the illustrations, RA stands for right arm, LA for left arm, RL for right leg, LL for left leg, C for chest, and G for ground.

Electrode positions

In the three- and five-leadwire systems, electrode positions for one lead may be identical to those for another lead. When that happens, change the lead selector switch to the setting that corresponds to the lead you want. In some cases, you'll need to reposition the electrodes.

Telemetry

In a telemetry monitoring system, you can create the same leads as the other systems with just two electrodes and a ground wire.

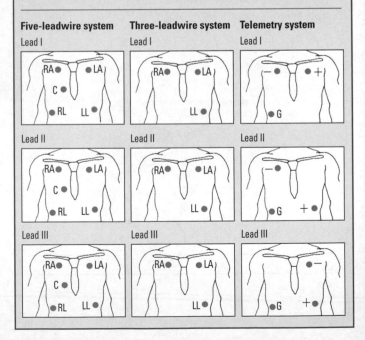

Five-leadwire system	Three-leadwire system	Telemetry system
Lead I	Lead I	Lead I
Lead II	Lead II	Lead II
Lead III	Lead III	Lead III

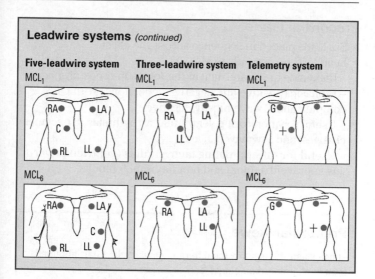

Leadwire systems *(continued)*

Five-leadwire system
MCL₁

Three-leadwire system
MCL₁

Telemetry system
MCL₁

MCL₆

MCL₆

MCL₆

Augmented unipolar leads

- Lead aV_R
  - Positive electrode on the right arm
  - Negative deflection
- Lead aV_L
  - Positive electrode on the left arm
  - Usually a positive deflection
- Lead aV_F
  - Positive electrode on the left leg
  - Positive deflection
  - Useful for monitoring the inferior wall of the left ventricle

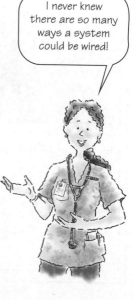

I never knew there are so many ways a system could be wired!

Precordial leads

- Six leads placed in sequence across the chest
- Lead V_1 (corresponds to MCL_1)
  – Right side of the sternum at the fourth intercostal space
  – Biphasic (positive and negative deflections) with QRS complex and T wave mostly negative
  – Useful for monitoring ventricular arrhythmias, ST-segment changes, and P-wave changes
  – Useful for differentiating tachycardias (ventricular versus supraventricular) and bundle-branch blocks

Precordial views

These illustrations show the different views of the heart obtained from each precordial (chest) lead.

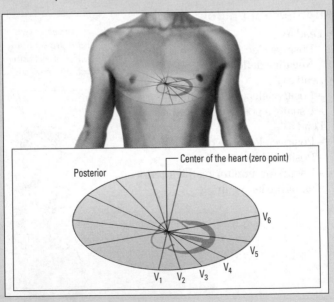

- Lead V_2
  - Left of the sternum at the fourth intercostal space
  - Negative deflection with a small amount of positive deflection
  - Useful for detecting ST-segment elevation
- Lead V_3
  - Between V_2 and V_4 at the fifth intercostal space
  - Biphasic (positive and negative deflections)
  - Useful for detecting ST-segment elevation
- Lead V_4
  - Fifth intercostal space at the midclavicular line
  - Positive deflection
  - Useful for detecting ST-segment and T-wave changes
- Lead V_5
  - Fifth intercostal space at the anterior axillary line
  - Positive deflection
  - Useful for detecting ST-segment and T-wave changes
- Lead V_6 (equivalent to MCL_6)
  - Fifth intercostal space at the midaxillary line
  - Positive deflection

Modified chest leads

- MCL_1 (the lead equivalent of V_1 on the 12-lead ECG)
  - Mostly negative deflection
  - Useful for assessing QRS-complex arrhythmias, monitoring premature ventricular beats and P-wave changes, distinguishing between different types of tachycardia (such as ventricular and supraventricular) and bundle-branch defects, and confirming pacemaker wire placement
- MCL_6 (alternative to MCL_1)
  - Same location as its equivalent, lead V_6
  - Positive deflection
  - Useful for monitoring ventricular conduction changes

ECG grid

- Waveforms produced by the heart's electrical current are recorded on ECG graphing paper.
- The horizontal axis of the ECG strip represents time.
  - Each small block equals 0.04 second.
  - Five small blocks form a large block, which equals 0.2 second (0.04 second [one small block] multiplied by 5 [small blocks in a large block] = 0.2 second).
  - Five large blocks equal 1 second (5 × 0.2).
  - To measure or calculate heart rate (in beats per minute), use a 6-second strip, which consists of 30 large blocks.

ECG grid

This ECG grid shows the horizontal and vertical axes and their respective measurement values.

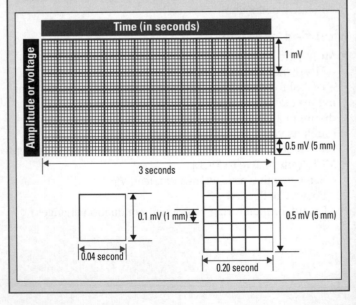

- The vertical axis of the ECG measures amplitude in millimeters (mm) or electrical voltage in millivolts (mV).
  – Each small block represents 1 mm or 0.1 mV.
  – Each large block represents 5 mm or 0.5 mV.
  – To determine the amplitude of an ECG component (wave, segment, or interval), count the number of small blocks from the baseline to the highest (in a positive wave) or lowest (in a negative wave) point of the wave, segment, or interval on a standard 12-lead ECG.

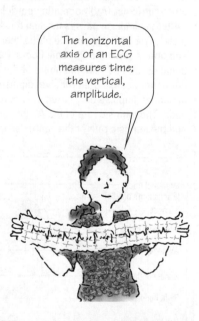

The horizontal axis of an ECG measures time; the vertical, amplitude.

ECG complex

- Represents electrical events occurring in one cardiac cycle
- Represents conduction of electrical impulses from the atria to the ventricles

Cardiac conduction system

The conduction system of the heart, shown below, begins with the heart's dominant pacemaker, the sinoatrial (SA) node. The intrinsic rate of the SA node is 60 to 100 beats/minute. When an impulse leaves the SA node, it travels through the atria along Bachmann's bundle and the internodal pathways on its way to the atrioventricular (AV) node and ventricles.

After the impulse passes through the AV node, it travels to the ventricles, first down the bundle of His, then along the bundle branches, and finally down the Purkinje fibers. Pacemaker cells in the junctional tissue and Purkinje fibers of the ventricles normally remain dormant because they receive impulses from the SA node. They initiate an impulse only when they don't receive one from the SA node. The intrinsic rate of the AV junction is 40 to 60 beats/minute, and the intrinsic rate of the ventricles is 20 to 40 beats/minute.

Interatrial tract (Bachmann's bundle)
SA node
Internodal tracts
AV node
Bundle of His (AV bundle)
Right bundle branch
Left bundle branch
Purkinje fibers

Through the ages

Pediatric pacemaker rates

In children younger than age 3, the AV node may discharge impulses at a rate of 50 to 80 times per minute; the Purkinje fibers may discharge at a rate of 40 to 50 times per minute.

- Consists of five waveforms labeled with the letters P, Q, R, S, and T
- Contains three elements (Q, R, and S) that form one unit, the QRS complex

ECG waveform components

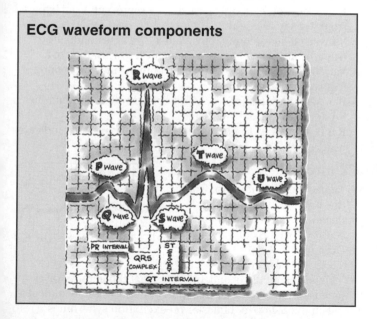

P wave

- Represents atrial depolarization or conduction of an electrical impulse through the atria
- Location: Precedes the QRS complex
- Amplitude: 2 to 3 mm
- Duration: 0.06 to 0.12 second
- Configuration: Usually rounded, upright
- Deflection:
  – Positive (upright) in leads I, II, aV_F, and V_2 to V_6
  – Usually positive but may vary in leads III and aV_L
  – Negative (inverted) in lead aV_R
  – Biphasic (variable) in lead V_1
- With normal deflection and configuration, electrical impulses most likely originate in the sinoatrial (SA) node
- If peaked, notched, or enlarged, may represent atrial hypertrophy or enlargement
- If inverted, may signify retrograde or reverse conduction from the atrioventricular (AV) junction toward the atria
- Varying P waves indicate that the impulse may be coming from different sites in the atria
- If absent, may signify conduction by a route other than the SA node
- If a P wave doesn't precede the QRS complex, may indicate heart block

PR interval

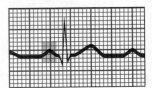

- Tracks the atrial impulse from the atria through the AV node
- Location: Start of the P wave to start of the QRS complex
- Duration:
  – 0.12 to 0.20 second
  – If less than 0.12 second, indicates that the impulse originated somewhere other than the SA node, possibly indicating junctional arrhythmias or preexcitation syndromes
  – If greater than 0.20 second, represents a conduction delay through the atria or AV junction

QRS complex

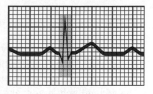

- Represents depolarization of and impulse conduction through the ventricles, after which the ventricles contract and blood is ejected and pumped through the arteries, creating a pulse
- Represents ventricular electrical activity but doesn't guarantee a mechanical contraction or a pulse (the contraction could be weak, as with premature ventricular contractions, or the contraction could be absent, as with pulseless electrical activity)
- Location: Follows the PR interval
- Amplitude: 5 to 30 mm, but differs for each lead used
- Duration:
  – 0.06 to 0.10 second, or one-half of the PR interval
  – Measured from the start of the Q wave to the end of the S wave or from the start of the R wave if the Q wave is absent
- Configuration:
  – Includes the Q wave (the first negative deflection, or deflection below the baseline, after the P wave), the R wave (the first positive deflection after the Q wave), and the S wave (the first negative deflection after the R wave)
  – May not display all three waves
  – Will look different in each lead
- Deflection:
  – Positive in leads I, II, III, aV_L, aV_F, and V_4 to V_6
  – Negative in leads aV_R and V_1 to V_2
  – Biphasic in lead V_3

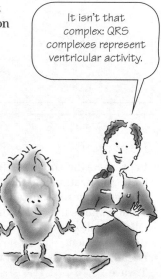

It isn't that complex: QRS complexes represent ventricular activity.

QRS waveform variety

The illustrations below show the various configurations of QRS complexes. When documenting a QRS complex, use uppercase letters to indicate a wave with a normal or high amplitude (greater than 5 mm) and lowercase letters to indicate one with a low amplitude (less than 5 mm).

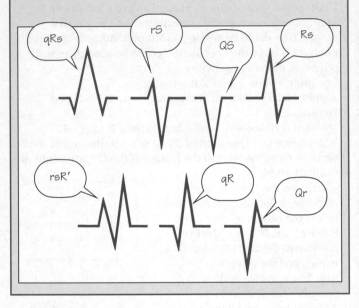

ST segment

- Represents the end of ventricular depolarization and the start of ventricular repolarization
- J point: Marks the end of the QRS complex and the start of the ST segment
- Location: From the end of the S wave to the start of the T wave

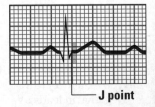

ST-segment changes

Closely monitoring the ST segment on a patient's ECG can help you detect myocardial ischemia or injury before infarction develops.

ST-segment depression

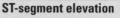

An ST segment is considered depressed when it's 0.5 mm or more below the baseline. A depressed ST segment may indicate myocardial ischemia or digoxin toxicity.

ST-segment elevation

An ST segment is considered elevated when it's 1 mm or more above the baseline. An elevated ST segment may indicate myocardial injury.

- Deflection:
  - Usually isoelectric (along the baseline, neither positive nor negative)
  - May vary from -0.5 to $+1$ mm in some precordial leads
- May become elevated or depressed

T *wave*

- Represents the relative refractory period of repolarization or ventricular recovery at peak
- Location: Follows the ST segment

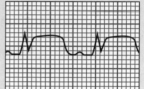

- Amplitude: 0.5 mm in leads I, II, and III and up to 10 mm in precordial leads
- Configuration: Typically rounded and smooth

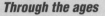

Through the ages

Older adult ECGs

Always keep the patient's age in mind when interpreting an ECG. An older adult's ECG may include increased PR, QRS, and QT intervals; decreased amplitude of the QRS complex; and a shift of the QRS axis to the left.

- Deflection:
  – Usually positive or upright in leads I, II, aV_L, aV_F, and V_2 to V_6
  – Inverted in lead aV_R
  – Variable in leads III and V_1
- If bumps appear in the T wave, may indicate hidden P wave
- If tall, peaked, or tented, may indicate myocardial injury or electrolyte imbalances (hyperkalemia)
- If inverted in leads I, II, aV_L, aV_F, or V_2 through V_6, may represent myocardial ischemia

QT interval

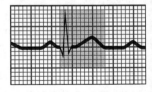

- Measures the time needed for ventricular depolarization and repolarization
- Location: The start of the QRS complex to the end of the T wave
- Duration:
  – Varies with age, sex, and heart rate
  – Lasts 0.36 to 0.44 second
  – When the rhythm is regular, shouldn't be greater than half the distance between two consecutive R waves

Drugs that increase the QT interval

This chart lists drugs that have been shown to increase the QT interval, which increases the patient's risk of developing torsades de points.

Drug name	Drug class	Drug name	Drug class
amiodarone	antiarrhythmic	halofantrine	antimalarial
arsenic trioxide	antineoplastic	haloperidol	antipsychotic
chloroquine	antimalarial	ibutilide	antiarrhythmic
chlorpromazine	antipsychotic/ antiemetic	levomethadyl	opiate agonist
		methadone	opiate agonist
clarithromycin	antibiotic	pentamidine	anti-infective
disopyramide	antiarrhythmic	pimozide	antipsychotic
dofetilide	antiarrhythmic	procainamide	antiarrhythmic
domperidone	antinauseant	quinidine	antiarrhythmic
droperidol	sedative; antinauseant	sotalol	antiarrhythmic
erythromycin	antibiotic; GI stimulant	thioridazine	antipsychotic

- If prolonged, indicates slowed ventricular repolarization, possibly from:
  – Effects of certain drugs (such as class I antiarrhythmics) or electrolyte imbalances (such as hypocalcemia)
  – Prolonged QT syndrome (a congenital conduction-system defect present in certain families)
- If shortened, may result from digoxin toxicity or electrolyte imbalances (such as hypercalcemia)

U wave

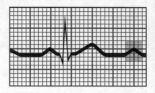

- Represents repolarization of the His-Purkinje system
- May not appear on ECG
- Location: Follows the T wave
- Configuration: Typically upright and rounded
- Deflection: Upright
- If prominent, may indicate hypercalcemia, hypokalemia, or digoxin toxicity

8-step method of ECG evaluation

Determine rhythm.
- Atrial rhythm:
  - Measure P-P intervals for several cycles.
  - If consistently similar, atrial rhythm is regular.
  - If dissimilar, atrial rhythm is irregular.
- Ventricular rhythm:
  - Measure the intervals between two consecutive R waves in the QRS complexes.
  - If no R wave, use the Q wave or

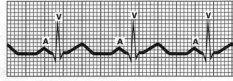

the S wave of consecutive QRS complexes.
  - If R-R intervals are consistently similar, ventricular rhythm is regular.
  - If dissimilar, ventricular rhythm is irregular.

Calculate rate using one of three methods: times-10; 1,500; or sequence.
- Times-10 method
  - Obtain a 6-second strip.
  - Count the number of P waves.
  - Multiply the number of P waves by 10 (ten 6-second strips equal 1 minute) to calculate the atrial rate.
  - Calculate ventricular rate the same way using R waves.
- 1,500 method (because 1,500 small squares equal 1 minute)
  - Count the number of small squares between identical points on two consecutive P waves.
  - Divide the number by 1,500 to get the atrial rate.
  - Use the same method with two consecutive R waves to cal-

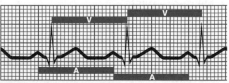

culate the ventricular rate.

- Sequence method
  - Find a P wave that peaks on a heavy black line.
  - Assign these numbers to the next six heavy black lines: 300, 150, 100, 75, 60, and 50.
  - Find the next P wave peak.
  - Estimate the atrial rate based on the number assigned to the nearest heavy black line.
  - Estimate the ventricular rate the same way using the R wave.

Evaluate P wave.

- Determine if a P wave is present for every QRS complex.
- Assess whether it has a normal configuration, size, and shape.

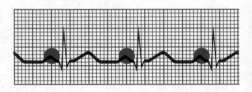

Determine PR interval duration.

- Count the small squares between the start of the P wave and the start of the QRS complex.

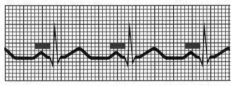

- Multiply the number of squares by 0.04 second.
- Determine if the duration is normal (0.12 to 0.20 second, or 3 to 5 small squares) and consistent.

Determine QRS complex duration.

- Measure straight across from the beginning of the QRS complex to the end of the S wave (not just to the peak).

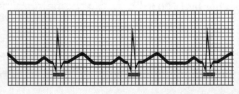

- Count the small squares between the beginning and end of the QRS complex.
- Multiply this number by 0.04 second.
- Determine if the duration is normal (0.06 to 0.10 second), all QRS complexes are the same size and shape, and a complex appears after every P wave.

Evaluate T wave.

- Determine if T waves are present and have a normal shape, normal amplitude, and the same deflection as the QRS complexes.

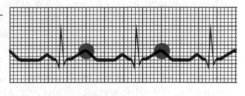

- Consider whether a P wave could be hidden in a T wave.

Determine QT interval duration.

- Count the small squares between the beginning of the QRS complex and the end of the T wave (where the T wave returns to the baseline).
- Multiply this number by 0.04 second.
- Determine if the duration is normal (0.36 to 0.44 second).

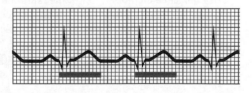

Evaluate other components.

- Make sure that the waveform doesn't reflect problems with the monitor.
- Note ectopic beats, aberrantly conducted beats, or other abnormalities.

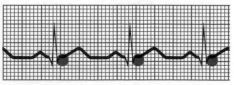

Methods of measuring rhythm

Paper-and-pencil method

- Place the ECG strip on a flat surface.
- Position the straight edge of a piece of paper along the strip's baseline.
- Move the paper up slightly so the straight edge is near the peak of the R wave.
- With a pencil, mark the paper at the R waves of two consecutive QRS complexes, as shown below. This is the R-R interval.
- Move the paper across the strip lining up the two marks with succeeding R-R intervals. If the distance for each R-R interval is the same, the ventricular rhythm is regular. If the distance varies, the rhythm is irregular.
- Use the same method to measure the distance between P waves (the P-P interval) and determine whether the atrial rhythm is regular or irregular.

Caliper method

- With the ECG on a flat surface, place one point of the calipers on the peak of the first R wave of two consecutive QRS complexes.
- Adjust the caliper legs so the other point is on the peak of the next R wave, as shown below. This distance is the R-R interval.
- Pivot the first point of the calipers toward the third R wave and note whether it falls on the peak of that wave.
- Check succeeding R-R intervals in the same way. If they're all the same, the ventricular rhythm is regular. If they vary, the rhythm is irregular.
- Using the same method, measure the P-P intervals to determine whether the atrial rhythm is regular or irregular.

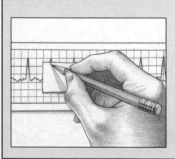

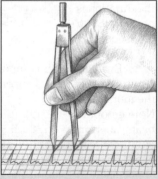

- Check the ST segment for abnormalities.
- Look for a U wave.
- Classify the rhythm strip according to one or all of the following characteristics:
  – Site of origin of the rhythm (sinus node, atria, AV node, or ventricles)
  – Rate (normal [60 to 100 beats/minute], bradycardic [less than 60 beats/minute], tachycardic [more than 100 beats/minute])
  – Rhythm (regular or irregular [flutter, fibrillation, heart block, escape rhythm, other arrhythmias]).

Make sure that the abnormalities you see on an ECG waveform aren't caused by monitor problems.

Correcting the QT interval

The QT interval is affected by the patient's heart rate. As the heart rate increases, the QT interval decreases; as the heart rate decreases, the QT interval increases. For this reason, evaluating the QT interval based on a standard heart rate of 60 is recommended. This corrected QT interval is known as QTc.

The following formula is used to determine the QTc:

$$\frac{QT\ interval}{\sqrt{R\text{-}R\ interval\ in\ seconds}}$$

The normal QTc for women is less than 0.46 second and for men is less than 0.45 second. When the QTc is longer than 0.50 second in men or women, torsades de pointes is more likely to develop.

(Text continues on page 32.)

Identifying monitor problems

Abnormal waveforms could indicate monitor problems. This chart reviews commonly encountered problems, their possible causes, and suggested interventions. Remember, however, you should always assess the patient before troubleshooting the equipment.

Waveform	Possible causes
Artifact *(waveform interference)* 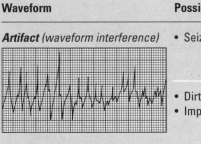	• Seizures, chills, or anxiety
	• Dirty or corroded connections • Improper electrode application
	• Short circuit in leadwires or cable
	• Electrical interference from other equipment in the room
	• Static electricity interference from inadequate room humidity
False-high-rate alarm 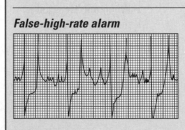	• Gain setting too high, particularly with MCL$_1$ setting
	• HIGH alarm set too low, or LOW alarm set too high

Interventions

• If the patient is having a seizure, notify the doctor and intervene as needed.
• Keep the patient warm and encourage relaxation.

• Replace dirty or corroded wires.
• Check the electrodes and reapply them if needed. Clean the patient's skin well because skin oils and dead skin cells inhibit conduction.
• Check the electrode gel. If it's dry, apply new electrodes.

• Replace broken equipment.

• Make sure all electrical equipment is attached to a common ground. Check all three-prong plugs to make sure no prongs are loose. Notify the biomedical engineering department.

• Regulate room humidity to 40% if possible.

• Assess the patient for evidence of hyperkalemia.
• Reset gain.

• Set alarm limits according to the patient's heart rate.

(continued)

Identifying monitor problems *(continued)*

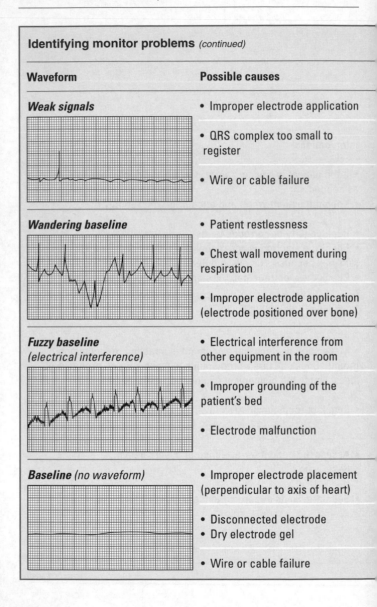

Waveform	Possible causes
Weak signals	• Improper electrode application
	• QRS complex too small to register
	• Wire or cable failure
Wandering baseline	• Patient restlessness
	• Chest wall movement during respiration
	• Improper electrode application (electrode positioned over bone)
Fuzzy baseline *(electrical interference)*	• Electrical interference from other equipment in the room
	• Improper grounding of the patient's bed
	• Electrode malfunction
Baseline *(no waveform)*	• Improper electrode placement (perpendicular to axis of heart)
	• Disconnected electrode
	• Dry electrode gel
	• Wire or cable failure

Interventions

• Reapply the electrodes.

• Reset gain so the height of the complex is more than 1 mV.
• Try monitoring the patient on another lead.

• Replace faulty wires or cables.

• Encourage the patient to relax.

• Make sure that tension on the cable isn't pulling the electrode away from the patient's body.

• Reposition improperly placed electrodes.

• Make sure all electrical equipment is attached to a common ground.
• Check all three-prong plugs to make sure no prongs are loose.

• Make sure the bed ground is attached to the room's common ground.

• Replace the electrodes.

• Reposition improperly placed electrodes.

• Check if electrodes are disconnected.
• Check electrode gel. If the gel is dry, apply new electrodes.

• Replace faulty wires or cables.

Normal sinus rhythm

- The standard against which all other rhythms are compared
- Represents an impulse that progresses from the SA node to the ventricles through the normal conduction pathway

Recognizing normal sinus rhythm

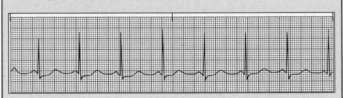

Rhythm
- Atrial regular
- Ventricular regular

Rate
- 60 to 100 beats/minute (SA node's normal firing rate)

P wave
- Normal shape (round and smooth)
- Upright in lead II
- One for every QRS complex
- All similar in size and shape

PR interval
- Within normal limits (0.12 to 0.20 second)

QRS complex
- Within normal limits (0.06 to 0.10 second)

T wave
- Normal shape
- Upright and rounded in lead II

QT interval
- Within normal limits (0.36 to 0.44 second)

Other
- No ectopic or aberrant beats

Sinus node arrhythmias

2

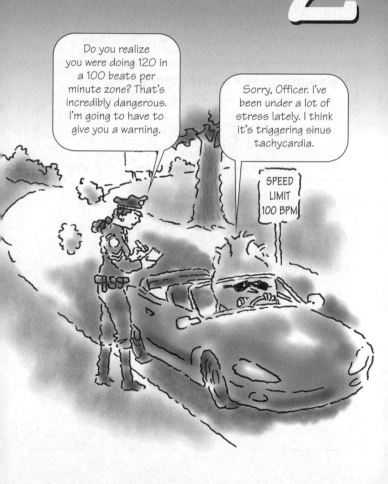

Sinus arrhythmia

- Rate usually within normal limits
- Rhythm irregular and corresponds to the respiratory cycle
- Occurs as the heart's normal response to respiration
- May be a normal finding in athletes, children, and older adults
- Rarely occurs in infants

What causes it

- Inhibition of reflex vagal activity (tone)
- Inferior-wall myocardial infarction (MI)

Recognizing sinus arrhythmia

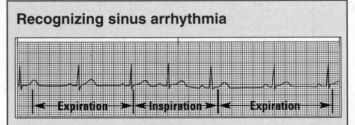

Rhythm
- Irregular
- Corresponds to the respiratory cycle
- P-P interval and R-R interval shorter during inspiration; longer during expiration
- Difference between longest and shortest P-P interval exceeds 0.12 second

Rate
- Usually within normal limits (60 to 100 beats/minute)
- Varies with respiration
- Increases during inspiration
- Decreases during expiration

P wave
- Normal size
- Normal configuration

PR interval
- May vary slightly
- Within normal limits

QRS complex
- Preceded by P wave

T wave
- Normal size
- Normal configuration

QT interval
- May vary slightly
- Usually within normal limits

Other
- Phasic slowing and quickening

- Drugs
  - Digoxin
  - Morphine
- Increased intracranial pressure (ICP)

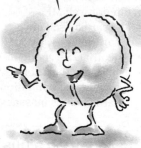

Drugs such as digoxin and morphine are just one possible cause of sinus arrhythmias.

During inspiration
- Increased venous return
- Decreased vagal tone
- Increased heart rate

During expiration
- Decreased venous return
- Increased vagal tone
- Decreased heart rate

What to look for
- Possibly no symptoms (commonly insignificant)
- Increased peripheral pulse rate during inspiration
- Decreased peripheral pulse rate during expiration
- Possible disappearance of arrhythmia when heart rate increases, such as during exercise
- Signs and symptoms of underlying condition, if present
- Dizziness or syncope (with marked sinus arrhythmia)

How it's treated
- If sinus arrhythmia develops suddenly in a patient who's taking digoxin, notify the doctor. The patient may have developed digoxin toxicity.
- Treatment usually isn't needed if the patient is asymptomatic.
- If unrelated to respiration (abnormal), treat the underlying cause.
- If induced by morphine, notify the doctor, who will decide whether to continue giving the drug.

Sinus bradycardia

- Rate less than 60 beats/minute
- Rhythm regular
- Impulses originating in the sinus node

What causes it

- Cardiomyopathy
- Heart block
- Inferior-wall MI
- Myocardial ischemia
- Myocarditis
- Sinoatrial (SA) node disease
- Conditions that increase vagal stimulation or decrease sympathetic stimulation
  - Carotid sinus massage

Recognizing sinus bradycardia

Rhythm
- Regular

Rate
- Less than 60 beats/minute

P wave
- Normal size
- Normal configuration
- P wave before each QRS complex

PR interval
- Within normal limits
- Constant

QRS complex
- Normal duration
- Normal configuration

T wave
- Normal size
- Normal configuration

QT interval
- Within normal limits
- Possibly prolonged

- – Deep relaxation
- – Sleep
- – Valsalva's maneuver
- – Vomiting
- Glaucoma
- Hyperkalemia
- Hypothermia
- Hypothyroidism
- Increased ICP
- Drugs
  - – Antiarrhythmics (amiodarone, propafenone, quinidine, sotalol)
  - – Beta-adrenergic blockers (metoprolol, propranolol)
  - – Calcium channel blockers (diltiazem, verapamil)
  - – Digoxin
  - – Lithium
- Possibly normal in well-conditioned athletes

What to look for
- Pulse rate less than 60 beats/minute
- Regular rhythm
- Possibly bradycardia-induced syncope (known as a *Stokes-Adams attack*)

If patient can compensate for decreased cardiac output
- No symptoms

If patient can't compensate
- Altered mental status
- Blurred vision
- Chest pain
- Cool, clammy skin
- Crackles
- Dizziness
- Dyspnea (shortness of breath)
- Hypotension
- S_3 heart sound, indicating heart failure
- Syncope

How it's treated

- Usually, no treatment is needed if the patient has stable vital signs and no symptoms.
- Continue to observe the patient's heart rhythm and monitor the progression and duration of bradycardia.
- Evaluate the patient's tolerance for the rhythm at rest and with activity.
- Review the patient's drug regimen.
- If the patient has symptoms of reduced cardiac output, identify and correct the underlying cause, if possible, and take steps to determine the proper treatment using a bradycardia algorithm. Prompt attention is critical. The heart of a patient with underlying cardiac disease may not be able to increase stroke volume to compensate for a decrease in rate. Notify the doctor immediately.

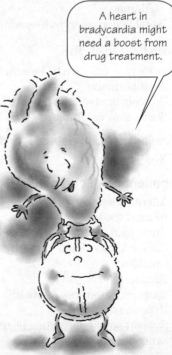

A heart in bradycardia might need a boost from drug treatment.

- Prepare the patient for treatments as needed, such as drug administration (atropine, dopamine, epinephrine); transvenous or transcutaneous pacing; or permanent pacemaker insertion for a chronic, symptomatic condition.

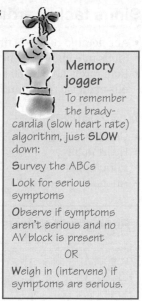

Memory jogger

To remember the brady-cardia (slow heart rate) algorithm, just **SLOW** down:

Survey the ABCs

Look for serious symptoms

Observe if symptoms aren't serious and no AV block is present

OR

Weigh in (intervene) if symptoms are serious.

Sinus tachycardia

- Accelerated SA node firing
- Sinus rate above 100 beats/minute in an adult
- Rate rarely above 160 beats/minute, except during strenuous exercise (maximum rate declines with age)

What causes it

- Cardiogenic shock
- Heart failure
- Pericarditis
- Anemia

Recognizing sinus tachycardia

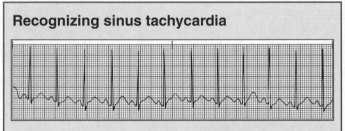

Rhythm
- Regular

Rate
- Greater than 100 beats/minute

P wave
- Normal size
- Normal configuration
- May increase in amplitude
- Precedes each QRS complex
- As heart rate increases, possibly superimposed on preceding T wave and difficult to identify

PR interval
- Within normal limits
- Constant

QRS complex
- Normal duration
- Normal configuration

T wave
- Normal size
- Normal configuration

QT interval
- Within normal limits
- Commonly shortened

- Hypovolemia
- Hemorrhage
- Hyperthyroidism
- Respiratory distress
- Pulmonary embolism
- Sepsis
- Drugs
  - Aminophylline
  - Amphetamines
  - Atropine
  - Dobutamine
  - Dopamine
  - Epinephrine
  - Isoproterenol
  - Nitrates
- Possibly normal response to:
  - Exercise
  - Fever
  - Pain
  - Stress
  - Strong emotions (fear, anxiety)

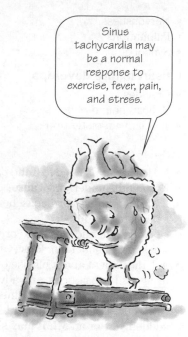

Sinus tachycardia may be a normal response to exercise, fever, pain, and stress.

Triggers

- Alcohol
- Caffeine
- Nicotine

What to look for

- Heart rate above 100 beats/minute
- Regular rhythm
- Typically no symptoms

If cardiac output falls and compensatory mechanisms fail

- Anxiety
- Blurred vision
- Chest pain
- Hypotension

- Nervousness
- Palpitations
- Syncope

If heart failure develops

- Crackles
- S_3 heart sound
- Jugular vein distention

How it's treated

- No treatment is needed if the patient is asymptomatic.
- Correct the underlying cause.
- If the patient has cardiac ischemia, give drugs to slow the heart rate, including:
  – beta-adrenergic blockers (propranolol or atenolol)
  – calcium channel blockers (verapamil or diltiazem).
- Ask the patient about his use of tachycardia-triggering drugs and substances, and advise abstinence from alcohol, caffeine, and nicotine.
- Notify the doctor promptly if sinus tachycardia arises suddenly after an MI. It may signal an extension of the infarct.
- Provide a calm environment, and help the patient with relaxation techniques.
- Help reduce the patient's fear and anxiety.

Sinus arrest

- Normal sinus rhythm maintained, with occasional, prolonged failure of SA node to initiate an impulse
- Episodic failure in automaticity or impulse formation of the SA node and lack of atrial stimulation
- PQRST complex or complexes missing

Recognizing sinus arrest

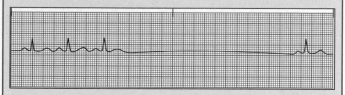

Rhythm
- Regular except during arrest (irregular as result of missing complexes)

Rate
- Usually within normal limits (60 to 100 beats/minute) before arrest
- Length or frequency of pause may result in bradycardia

P wave
- Periodically absent, with entire PQRST complexes missing
- When present, normal size and configuration
- Precedes each QRS complex

PR interval
- Within normal limits when a P wave is present

- Constant when a P wave is present

QRS complex
- Normal duration
- Normal configuration
- Absent during arrest

T wave
- Normal size
- Normal configuration
- Absent during arrest

QT interval
- Within normal limits
- Absent during arrest

Other
- The pause isn't a multiple of the underlying P-P intervals
- Junctional escape beats may occur at end of pause

What causes it

- Acute inferior-wall MI
- Acute myocarditis
- Cardiomyopathy
- Coronary artery disease (CAD)
- Hypertensive heart disease
- Acute infection
- Sick sinus syndrome
- Increased vagal tone or carotid sinus sensitivity
- Sinus node disease
- Cardioactive drugs
  - Amiodarone
  - Beta-adrenergic blockers (bisoprolol, metoprolol, propranolol)
  - Calcium channel blockers (diltiazem, verapamil)
  - Digoxin
  - Quinidine
  - Procainamide
  - Salicylate toxicity

What to look for

- Absence of heart sounds and pulse during arrest
- Absence of symptoms with short pauses
- Evidence of decreased cardiac output with recurrent or prolonged pauses
  - Low blood pressure
  - Altered mental status
  - Cool, clammy skin
  - Syncope or near-syncope
  - Dizziness
  - Blurred vision

How it's treated

- No treatment is needed if the patient is asymptomatic.
- If the patient has symptoms, follow the guidelines outlined in the bradycardia algorithm on page 266.

- As needed, discontinue drugs that affect SA node discharge or conduction, such as:
  - beta-adrenergic blockers
  - calcium channel blockers
  - digoxin.
- Protect the patient from the risk of injury, such as a fall, which may result from syncopal or near-syncopal episodes caused by a prolonged pause.

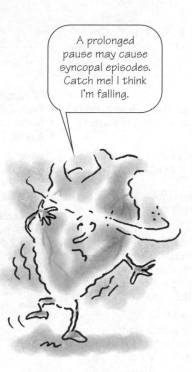

Sinoatrial exit block

- Regular discharges of the SA node
- Delayed or blocked SA node impulses with long sinus pauses
- Pause of indefinite length ending with sinus rhythm
- Possible lack of atrial activity

Recognizing sinoatrial exit block

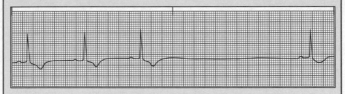

Rhythm
- Regular except during pause (irregular as result of pause)

Rate
- Usually within normal limits (60 to 100 beats/minute) before pause
- Length or frequency of pause may result in bradycardia

P wave
- Periodically absent, with entire PQRST complex missing
- When present, normal size and configuration and precedes each QRS complex

PR interval
- Within normal limits
- Constant when a P wave is present

QRS complex
- Normal duration
- Normal configuration
- Absent during a pause

T wave
- Normal size
- Normal configuration
- Absent during a pause

QT interval
- Within normal limits
- Absent during a pause

Other
- The pause is a multiple of the underlying P-P interval
- Sinus beat usually occurs at end of pause

What causes it

- Acute inferior-wall MI
- Acute myocarditis
- Cardiomyopathy
- CAD
- Hypertensive heart disease
- Acute infection
- Sick sinus syndrome
- Sinus node disease
- Increased vagal tone
- Salicylate toxicity
- Cardioactive drugs
  - Amiodarone
  - Beta-adrenergic blockers (bisoprolol, metoprolol, propranolol)
  - Calcium channel blockers (diltiazem, verapamil)
  - Digoxin
  - Quinidine
  - Procainamide

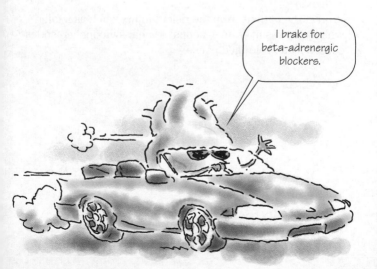

What to look for

- Absence of heart sounds and pulse during SA exit block
- Absence of symptoms with short pauses
- Evidence of decreased cardiac output with recurrent or prolonged pauses
  - Altered mental status
  - Blurred vision
  - Cool, clammy skin
  - Dizziness
  - Low blood pressure
  - Syncope or near-syncope

How it's treated

- No treatment is needed if the patient is asymptomatic.
- If the patient has symptoms, follow the guidelines outlined in the bradycardia algorithm on page 266.
- As needed, discontinue drugs that affect SA node discharge or conduction, such as:
  - beta-adrenergic blockers
  - calcium channel blockers
  - digoxin.
- Protect the patient from the risk of injury, such as a fall, which may result from syncopal or near-syncopal episodes caused by a prolonged pause.

Sick sinus syndrome

- Also known as *SA syndrome, sinus nodal dysfunction,* and *Stokes-Adams syndrome*
- Includes many SA node arrhythmias

What causes it

- Conditions that affect the atrial wall around the SA node by causing inflammation or degeneration of atrial tissue, which may lead to exit blocks

Recognizing sick sinus syndrome

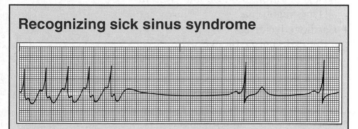

Rhythm
- Irregular
- Sinus pauses
- Abrupt rate changes

Rate
- Fast, slow, or alternating
- Interrupted by a long sinus pause

P wave
- Varies with rhythm changes
- May be normal size and configuration
- May be absent
- Usually precedes each QRS complex

PR interval
- Usually within normal limits
- Varies with rhythm changes

QRS complex
- Duration within normal limits
- Varies with rhythm changes
- Normal configuration

T wave
- Normal size
- Normal configuration

QT interval
- Usually within normal limits
- Varies with rhythm changes

Other
- Usually more than one arrhythmia on a 6-second strip

- Conditions leading to fibrosis of the SA node
  - Advanced age
  - Atherosclerotic heart disease
  - Cardiomyopathy
  - Hypertension
- Trauma to the SA node
  - Open-heart surgery, especially valve surgery
  - Pericarditis
  - Rheumatic heart disease
- Autonomic disturbances that affect autonomic innervation
  - Degeneration of autonomic system
  - Hypervagotonia
- Cardioactive drugs
  - Beta-adrenergic blockers
  - Calcium channel blockers
  - Digoxin

What to look for

- Fast, slow, or normal pulse rate
- Regular or irregular rhythm
- No increase in heart rate with exertion
- Episodes of tachy-brady syndrome, atrial flutter, atrial fibrillation, SA block, or sinus arrest

If underlying cardiomyopathy is present

- Dilated and displaced left ventricular apical impulse
- Possible crackles
- S_3 heart sound

If thromboembolism is present

- Acute pain
- Blurred vision
- Chest pain
- Dyspnea
- Fatigue
- Hypotension

- Neurologic changes (confusion, vision disturbances, weakness)
- Syncope (Stokes-Adams attacks)
- Tachycardia
- Tachypnea

How it's treated

- No treatment is needed if the patient is asymptomatic.
- If symptoms develop, alleviate them and correct the underlying cause.
- If the patient has symptoms, follow the guidelines outlined in the bradycardia algorithm on page 266.
- Prepare the patient for a temporary pacemaker (transcutaneous or transvenous).
- If the arrhythmia results from a chronic disorder, treatment may consist of digoxin, a beta-adrenergic blocker, or radio-frequency ablation. A permanent pacemaker may be inserted to maintain heart rate and ensure adequate cardiac output.
- Administer an anticoagulant for atrial fibrillation because of the risk of thromboembolic complications.
- Monitor the patient after starting beta-adrenergic blockers, calcium channel blockers, or other antiarrhythmics.

Through the ages

Mental status check

Because an older adult with sick sinus syndrome may have an altered mental status, be sure to perform a thorough assessment to rule out such disorders as stroke, delirium, or dementia.

Atrial arrhythmias

3

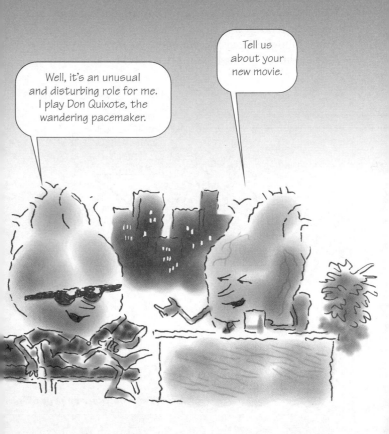

Premature atrial contractions

- Impulses originate in the atria, outside the sinoatrial (SA) node
  - From a single ectopic focus or multiple atrial foci that supersede the SA node as pacemaker for one or more beats
- May be conducted or nonconducted (blocked) through the atrioventricular (AV) node depending on the status of the AV node and the intraventricular conduction system
- Conducted premature atrial contractions (PACs)
  - Usually characterized by normal ventricular conduction
- Nonconducted PACs
  - Aren't followed by a QRS complex
  - May be difficult to distinguish from SA block

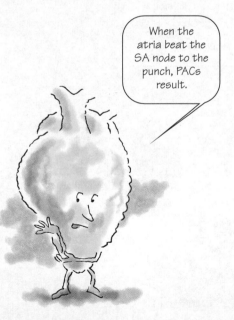

When the atria beat the SA node to the punch, PACs result.

(Text continues on page 57.)

Recognizing PACs

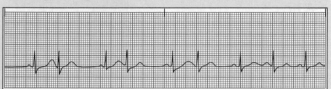

Rhythm
- Atrial: Irregular
- Ventricular: Irregular
- Underlying: Possibly regular

Rate
- Atrial and ventricular: Vary with underlying rhythm

P wave
- Premature
- Abnormal configuration compared to a sinus P wave
- If varying configurations, multiple ectopic sites
- May be hidden in preceding T wave

PR interval
- Usually within normal limits
- May be shortened or slightly prolonged for the ectopic beat, depending on the origin of ectopic focus

QRS complex
- Conducted: Duration and configuration usually normal
- Nonconducted: No QRS complex follows PAC

T wave
- Usually normal
- May be distorted if P wave is hidden in T wave

QT interval
- Usually within normal limits

Other
- May be a single beat
- May be bigeminal (every other beat premature)
- May be trigeminal (every third beat premature)
- May be quadrigeminal (every fourth beat premature)
- May occur in couplets (pairs)
- Three or more PACs in a row indicate atrial tachycardia

Distinguishing nonconducted PACs from SA block

To differentiate between nonconducted PACs and SA block, follow these guidelines:

• Whenever you see a pause in a rhythm, look carefully for a nonconducted P wave, which may occur before, during, or just after the T wave that precedes the pause.

• Compare the T wave that precedes the pause with other T waves on the rhythm strip. Look for slope distortion or an abnormality in its height or shape. These clues indicate where a nonconducted P wave may be hidden.

• If you find a P wave in the pause, check to see whether it's premature or whether it occurs earlier than subsequent sinus P waves. If it's premature (see the shaded area in the top rhythm strip below), it's a nonconducted PAC.

• If a P wave occurs in the pause or T wave (see the shaded area in the bottom rhythm strip below), then the rhythm represents SA block.

Nonconducted PAC

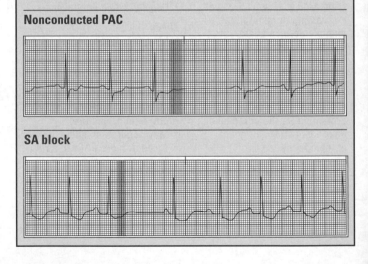

SA block

What causes it

- Enhanced automaticity in atrial tissue (most common cause)
- Coronary heart disease
- Valvular heart disease
- Heart failure
- Acute respiratory failure
- Chronic obstructive pulmonary disease (COPD)
- Hypoxia
- Digoxin toxicity
- Drugs that prolong absolute refractory period of SA node
  – Quinidine
  – Procainamide
- Electrolyte imbalances
- Endogenous catecholamine release from pain or anxiety
- Hyperthyroidism
- Anxiety
- Fatigue
- Fever
- Infectious disease

Triggers

- Alcohol
- Caffeine
- Nicotine

What to look for

- Pulse rhythm and rate that
  reflect the underlying rhythm
- Irregular peripheral or apical
  pulse rhythm when PACs
  occur
- Evidence of decreased cardiac
  output, such as hypotension
  and syncope, if the patient
  has heart disease

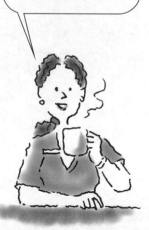

Common habits,
such as caffeine and
alcohol consumption,
can trigger many types
of atrial arrhythmias.

How it's treated

- Usually, no treatment is needed if the patient has no symptoms.
- If the patient has symptoms, treatment may focus on eliminating or controlling trigger factors, such as caffeine or alcohol consumption.
- Frequent PACs may be treated with drugs that prolong the atrial refractory period, such as beta-adrenergic blockers or calcium channel blockers.
- Patient teaching should be individually tailored to each patient.
  – Correct or avoid underlying causes or triggers, such as caffeine use.
  – Stress-reduction techniques may be taught to lessen anxiety.
- If the patient has ischemic or valvular heart disease, watch for evidence of heart failure, electrolyte imbalances, and more severe atrial arrhythmias. *Note:* In a patient with acute myocardial infarction (MI), PACs may be early signs of heart failure or an electrolyte imbalance.

Atrial tachycardia

- Supraventricular tachycardia (impulses originate above the ventricles)
- Atrial rate: 150 to 250 beats/minute
- Three forms

Atrial tachycardia with block

Multifocal atrial tachycardia (MAT, or *chaotic atrial rhythm*)

Paroxysmal atrial tachycardia (PAT), a transient event that starts and stops suddenly

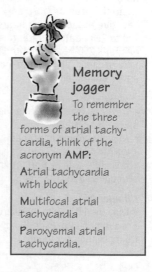

Memory jogger

To remember the three forms of atrial tachycardia, think of the acronym **AMP:**

Atrial tachycardia with block

Multifocal atrial tachycardia

Paroxysmal atrial tachycardia.

Recognizing atrial tachycardia

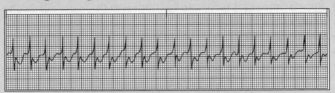

Rhythm
• Atrial: Usually regular
• Ventricular: Regular or irregular depending on AV conduction ratio and type of atrial tachycardia

Rate
• Atrial: Three or more consecutive ectopic atrial beats at 150 to 250 beats/minute; rarely exceeds 250 beats/minute
• Ventricular: Varies, depending on AV conduction ratio

P wave
• Deviates from normal appearance
• May be hidden in preceding T wave
• If visible, usually upright and precedes each QRS complex

PR interval
• May be difficult to measure if P wave can't be distinguished from preceding T wave

QRS complex
• Usually normal duration and configuration
• May be abnormal if impulses conducted abnormally through ventricles

T wave
• Usually visible
• May be distorted by P wave
• May be inverted if ischemia is present

QT interval
• Usually within normal limits
• May be shorter because of rapid rate

Other
• May be difficult to differentiate atrial tachycardia with block from sinus arrhythmia with U waves

Types of atrial tachycardia

Atrial tachycardia with block

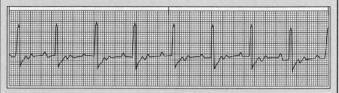

Rhythm
• Atrial: Regular
• Ventricular: Regular if block is constant, irregular if block is variable

Rate
• Atrial: 150 to 250 beats/minute
• Ventricular: Varies with block

P wave
• Slightly abnormal

PR interval
• Usually constant for conducted P waves
• May vary

QRS complex
• Usually normal

T wave
• Usually indiscernible

QT interval
• May be indiscernible

Other
• More than one P wave for each QRS complex

(continued)

What causes it

- Digoxin toxicity (most common cause)
- Cardiomyopathy
- MI
- Valvular heart disease
- Wolff-Parkinson-White (WPW) syndrome
- Cor pulmonale
- Systemic hypertension
- COPD

Types of atrial tachycardia *(continued)*

Multifocal atrial tachycardia

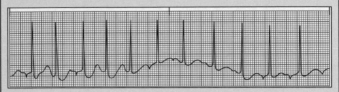

Rhythm
- Atrial: Irregular
- Ventricular: Irregular

Rate
- Atrial: 100 to 250 beats/minute (usually less than 160 beats/minute)
- Ventricular: 100 to 250 beats/minute

P wave
- Configuration: Varies
- Usually at least three different P wave shapes must appear

PR interval
- Varies

QRS complex
- Usually normal
- May become aberrant if arrhythmia persists

T wave
- Usually distorted

QT interval
- May be indiscernible

- Drugs
  - Albuterol
  - Cocaine
  - Marijuana
  - Theophylline
- Electrolyte imbalances
- Hypoxia
- Physical or psychological stress
- Congenital anomalies
- Hyperthyroidism

Types of atrial tachycardia *(continued)*

Paroxysmal atrial tachycardia

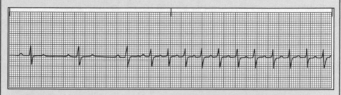

Rhythm
- Atrial: Regular
- Ventricular: Regular

Rate
- Atrial: 150 to 250 beats/minute
- Ventricular: 150 to 250 beats/minute

P wave
- May not be visible
- May be difficult to distinguish from preceding T wave

PR interval
- May not be measurable if P wave can't be distinguished from preceding T wave

QRS complex
- May be aberrantly conducted

T wave
- Usually indistinguishable

QT interval
- May be indistinguishable

Other
- Sudden onset, typically started by PAC; may start and stop abruptly

Triggers
- Alcohol
- Caffeine
- Nicotine

What to look for
- Rapid heart rate
- Regular or irregular rhythm, depending on type of atrial tachycardia
- Sudden feeling of palpitations, especially with PAT

- Decreased cardiac output and possible hypotension, chest pain, and syncope from persistent tachycardia and rapid ventricular rate, which leads to decreased ventricular filling time, increased myocardial oxygen consumption, and decreased oxygen supply to the myocardium
- Serious ventricular arrhythmias, especially if the patient has heart disease

How it's treated

- Treatment depends on the type of tachycardia and the severity of symptoms. It's directed toward eliminating the cause and decreasing the ventricular rate.
- Inquire about digoxin use, assess the patient for evidence of digoxin toxicity, and monitor digoxin blood levels.
- Valsalva's maneuver or carotid sinus massage may be used to treat PAT. If vagal maneuvers are used, keep resuscitative equipment readily available because vagal stimulation can cause bradycardia, ventricular arrhythmias, and asystole.
- Drug therapy (pharmacologic cardioversion) may be used to increase the degree of AV block and decrease the ventricular response rate. Appropriate drugs include:
  – adenosine
  – amiodarone
  – beta-adrenergic blockers

Through the ages

Stop sign for carotid sinus massage

Because carotid bruits may be absent, even with significant disease, carotid atherosclerosis might go undiagnosed in older adults. As a result, cardiac sinus massage shouldn't be performed in late middle-age and older patients. Embolic stroke may result if carotid massage is performed on a patient with significant atherosclerosis.

    – calcium channel blockers
    – digoxin.
- If other treatments fail or if the patient is unstable, synchronized electrical cardioversion may be used.
- Atrial overdrive pacing may stop the arrhythmia by suppressing spontaneous depolarization of the ectopic pacemaker with a series of paced electrical impulses.
- If the arrhythmia is related to WPW syndrome, catheter ablation may be used to control recurrent episodes of PAT.
- In patients with chronic pulmonary disease, treatment is directed at correcting hypoxia and electrolyte imbalances. The rhythm may not respond to antiarrhythmic drug treatment.

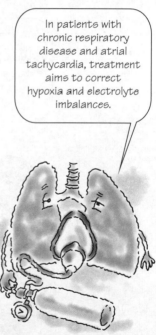

In patients with chronic respiratory disease and atrial tachycardia, treatment aims to correct hypoxia and electrolyte imbalances.

Atrial flutter

- A supraventricular tachycardia
- Atrial rate: 250 to 400 beats/minute (usually about 300 beats/minute)
- Originates in a single atrial focus
- Results from a reentrant circuit and possibly increased automaticity

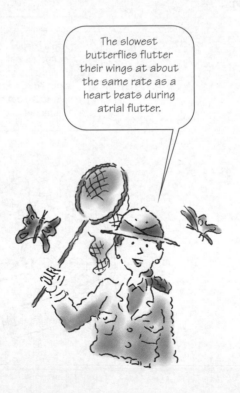

The slowest butterflies flutter their wings at about the same rate as a heart beats during atrial flutter.

Recognizing atrial flutter

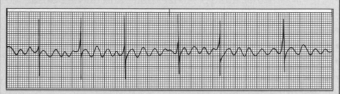

Rhythm
- Atrial: Regular
- Ventricular: Typically regular, although cycles may alternate (depends on AV conduction pattern)

Rate
- Atrial: 250 to 400 beats/minute
- Ventricular: Usually 60 to 100 beats/minute (one-half to one-fourth of atrial rate) but may be 125 to 150 beats/minute depending on the degree of AV block
- Usually expressed as a ratio (2:1 or 4:1, for example)
- Commonly 150 beats/minute ventricular and 300 beats/minute atrial, known as *2:1 block*
- Only every second, third, or fourth impulse is conducted to ventricles because the AV node usually won't accept more than 180 impulses/minute
- When atrial flutter is first recognized, ventricular rate typically exceeds 100 beats/minute

P wave
- Abnormal
- Sawtooth appearance known as *flutter waves* or *F waves*

PR interval
- Not measurable

QRS complex
- Duration: Usually within normal limits
- May be widened if flutter waves are buried within the complex

T wave
- Not identifiable

QT interval
- Not measurable because T wave isn't identifiable

Other
- Atrial rhythm may vary between a fibrillatory line and flutter waves (called *atrial fib-flutter*), with an irregular ventricular response
- May be difficult to differentiate atrial flutter from atrial fibrillation

What causes it

- Conditions that enlarge atrial tissue and elevate atrial pressures
- MI
- Cardiac surgery with acute MI
- COPD
- Hyperthyroidism
- Pericardial disease
- Primary myocardial disease
- Systemic arterial hypoxia
- Mitral valve disease
- Tricuspid valve disease
- Digoxin toxicity

What to look for

- Possibly no symptoms if ventricular rate is normal
- Rapid heart rate if ventricular rate is rapid (patient may complain of palpitations)
- Evidence of reduced cardiac output if ventricular rate is rapid
- Evidence of reduced ventricular filling time and coronary perfusion from rapid ventricular rate
  - Angina
  - Heart failure
  - Hypotension
  - Pulmonary edema
  - Syncope

How it's treated

- Interventions depend on the patient's cardiac function, preexcitation syndromes, and the duration of the arrhythmia (less or more than 48 hours).
- If the patient is hemodynamically unstable and atrial flutter has lasted 48 hours or less, synchronized electrical cardioversion or countershock should be performed immediately.

- If atrial flutter has lasted more than 48 hours, electrical cardioversion shouldn't be performed unless the patient is adequately anticoagulated because of the increased risk of thromboembolism. Anticoagulation therapy should be given before and after cardioversion.
- Keep resuscitative equipment at the bedside and stay alert for bradycardia because cardioversion can decrease the heart rate.
- In patients with otherwise normal heart function, administer a beta-adrenergic blocker, such as metoprolol, or a calcium channel blocker, such as diltiazem, to control the ventricular rate.
- In patients with impaired heart function (heart failure or ejection fraction less than 40%), use digoxin or amiodarone to control the ventricular rate.
- Stay alert to the effects of digoxin, which depresses the SA node.
- Because atrial flutter may reflect cardiac disease, monitor the patient closely for evidence of low cardiac output.
- Recurrent atrial flutter may be treated with ablation therapy.

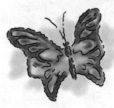

Atrial fibrillation

- Chaotic, asynchronous, electrical activity in atrial tissue
- Results from firing of multiple impulses from numerous ectopic pacemakers in the atria
- Absence of P waves
- Irregularly irregular ventricular response
- May be preceded by PACs

Recognizing atrial fibrillation

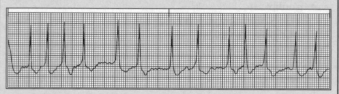

Rhythm
- Atrial: Irregularly irregular
- Ventricular: Irregularly irregular

Rate
- Atrial: Almost indiscernible, usually above 400 beats/minute; far exceeds ventricular rate because most impulses aren't conducted through the AV junction
- Ventricular: Usually 100 to 150 beats/minute but can be below 100 beats/minute

P wave
- Absent
- Replaced by baseline fibrillatory waves that represent atrial tetanization from rapid atrial depolarizations

PR interval
- Indiscernible

QRS complex
- Duration and configuration usually normal

T wave
- Indiscernible

QT interval
- Not measurable

Other
- Atrial rhythm may vary between fibrillatory line and flutter waves, called *atrial fib-flutter*
- It may be difficult to differentiate atrial fibrillation from atrial flutter and MAT

What causes it

- Acute MI
- Atrial septal defect
- Cardiomyopathy
- Coronary artery disease
- Hypertension
- Pericarditis
- Valvular heart disease (especially mitral valve disease)
- Rheumatic heart disease
- Cardiac surgery
- COPD
- Drugs such as aminophylline
- Digoxin toxicity
- Endogenous catecholamine released during exercise
- Hyperthyroidism

Triggers

- Alcohol
- Caffeine
- Nicotine

What to look for

- Irregularly irregular pulse rhythm with normal or abnormal heart rate
- Radial pulse rate that's slower than the apical pulse rate
- Palpable peripheral pulse only with stronger contractions, not with weaker ones that occur with atrial fibrillation
- Evidence of decreased end-diastolic volume (by about 20%) from loss of atrial kick,

decreased diastolic filling time from rapid heart rate, and decreased cardiac output:
– Light-headedness, syncope, and hypotension with new-onset atrial fibrillation and a rapid ventricular rate
• Possibly no symptoms with chronic atrial fibrillation, in which the patient may be able to compensate for decreased cardiac output, but an increased risk of pulmonary, cerebral, or other thromboembolic events

How it's treated
• Interventions aim to control the ventricular rate, establish anticoagulation, and restore and maintain a sinus rhythm.
• Treatment typically includes drug therapy to control the ventricular response or a combination of electrical cardioversion and drug therapy.
• If the patient is hemodynamically unstable, synchronized electrical cardioversion should be performed immediately. It's most successful if done within 48 hours after atrial fibrillation starts.
• If atrial fibrillation has lasted longer than 48 hours, electrical cardioversion shouldn't be performed unless the patient is adequately anticoagulated because of the risk of thromboembolism.
– If a thrombus forms in the atria, the resumption of normal contractions can result in systemic emboli.
– Anticoagulation therapy is crucial in reducing the risk of thromboembolism. Warfarin and heparin are used for anticoagulation before and after elective cardioversion.
– A transesophageal echocardiogram may be obtained before cardioversion to rule out thrombi in the atria.
• In patients with otherwise normal heart function, administer a beta-adrenergic blocker, such as metoprolol; a cardiac glycoside, such as digoxin; or a calcium channel blocker, such as diltiazem, to control the ventricular rate.
• In patients with impaired heart function (heart failure or ejection fraction less than 40%), use digoxin or amiodarone to control the ventricular rate.

(Text continues on page 75.)

Distinguishing atrial fibrillation from atrial flutter

It isn't uncommon for atrial flutter to have an irregular pattern of impulse conduction to the ventricles. In some leads, this pattern may be confused with atrial fibrillation. Here's how to tell the two arrhythmias apart.

Atrial fibrillation

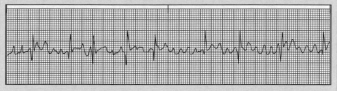

• Remember that fibrillatory waves (f waves) occur in an irregular pattern, making the atrial rhythm irregular.
• If you see atrial activity on the rhythm strip that, in some places, looks like flutter waves and seems to be regular for a short time and, in other places, looks like fibrillatory waves, interpret the rhythm as atrial fibrillation. Coarse fibrillatory waves sometimes have the characteristic sawtooth appearance of flutter waves.

Atrial flutter

• Look for characteristic abnormal P waves that produce a sawtooth appearance, known as flutter waves (F waves). These can be identified most easily in leads I, II, and V_1.

• Remember that the atrial rhythm is regular. You should be able to map the F waves across the rhythm strip. Although some F waves may occur within the QRS or T waves, other F waves are visible and occur on time.

Distinguishing atrial fibrillation from MAT

On an ECG, atrial fibrillation may look a lot like MAT. To determine whether a rhythm is atrial fibrillation or the similar MAT, focus on the P waves and the atrial and ventricular rhythms. You may find it helpful to look at a rhythm strip that's longer than 6 seconds.

Atrial fibrillation

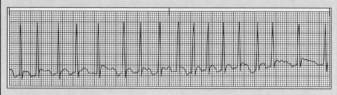

• Carefully look for discernible P waves before each QRS complex.
• If you can't clearly identify P waves and if fibrillatory waves appear in place of P waves, then the rhythm is probably atrial fibrillation.

• Carefully look at the rhythm, focusing on the R-R intervals. One of the hallmarks of atrial fibrillation is an irregularly irregular rhythm.

MAT

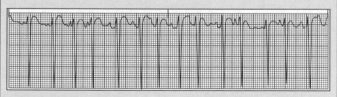

• P waves are present in MAT. Keep in mind, though, that at least three different P-wave shapes are visible in a single rhythm strip.
• You should be able to see most or all of the P-wave shapes repeat.

• Although the atrial and ventricular rhythms are irregular, the irregularity usually isn't as pronounced as it is in atrial fibrillation.

- Symptomatic atrial fibrillation that doesn't respond to routine treatment may be treated with radio-frequency ablation therapy.
- Monitor the apical and peripheral pulses; watch for evidence of decreased cardiac output and heart failure. If the patient isn't on a cardiac monitor, stay alert for an irregular pulse and differences in the radial and apical pulse rates.
- If drug therapy is used, monitor serum drug levels and watch for evidence of toxicity.
- Tell the patient to report changes in pulse rate, dizziness, faintness, chest pain, and signs of heart failure, such as dyspnea and peripheral edema.

Risk of restoring sinus rhythm

A patient with atrial fibrillation is at increased risk for developing an atrial thrombus and a systemic arterial embolism. Because the atria don't contract together in atrial fibrillation, blood may pool on the atrial wall and mural thrombi can form. Thrombus formation places the patient at higher risk for emboli and stroke.

When normal sinus rhythm is restored and the atria contract normally, clots can break away and travel through the pulmonary or systemic circulation, resulting in stroke or arterial occlusion.

Ashman's phenomenon

- Benign phenomenon characterized by aberrant conduction of premature supraventricular beats to the ventricles
- Commonly occurs with atrial fibrillation but may occur with any arrhythmia that affects the R-R interval
- Abnormal beat that usually occurs as right bundle-branch block (right bundle branch has slightly longer refractory period than the left does, so premature beats more commonly reach the right bundle when it's partly or fully refractory)

Ashman's phenomenon

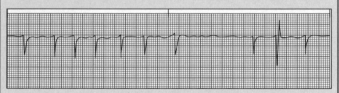

Rhythm
- Atrial: Irregular
- Ventricular: Irregular

Rate
- Reflects the underlying rhythm

P wave
- May be visible
- Abnormal configuration
- Unchanged if present in the underlying rhythm

PR interval
- Commonly changes on the premature beat, if measurable at all

QRS complex
- Altered configuration with right bundle-branch block pattern

T wave
- Deflection opposite that of QRS complex in most leads because of right bundle-branch block

QT interval
- Usually changed because of right bundle-branch block

Other
- No compensatory pause after an aberrant beat
- Aberrancy may continue for several beats and typically ends a short cycle preceded by a long cycle

What causes it

- A prolonged refractory period in a slower rhythm
- A short cycle followed by a long cycle because the refractory period varies with the length of the cycle

What to look for

- No signs or symptoms

How it's treated

- No interventions are needed for Ashman's phenomenon, although they may be needed for accompanying arrhythmias.

Phenomenal! Patients with Ashman's phenomenon typically present with no signs and symptoms and may not require treatment.

Wandering pacemaker

- Also called *wandering atrial pacemaker*
- A shifting site of impulse formation from the SA node to another area above the ventricles — the atria or AV junctional tissue
- May be normal in young patients
- Is common in athletes with slow heart rates

Recognizing wandering pacemaker

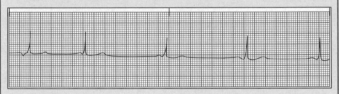

Rhythm
- Atrial: Varies slightly, with an irregular P-P interval
- Ventricular: Varies slightly, with an irregular R-R interval

Rate
- Varies, but usually within normal limits or less than 60 beats/minute

P wave
- Altered size and configuration from changing pacemaker site with at least three different P-wave shapes visible
- May be absent or inverted or occur after QRS complex if impulse originates in the AV junction

PR interval
- Varies from beat to beat as pacemaker site changes
- Usually less than 0.20 second
- Less than 0.12 second if the impulse originates in the AV junction

QRS complex
- Duration and configuration usually normal because ventricular depolarization is normal

T wave
- Normal size and configuration

QT interval
- Usually within normal limits

Other
- May be difficult to differentiate wandering pacemaker from PACs

Distinguishing wandering pacemaker from PACs

Because PACs are common, you may miss a wandering pacemaker rhythm unless you examine the rhythm strip carefully. You may find it helpful to look at a rhythm strip that's longer than 6 seconds.

Wandering pacemaker

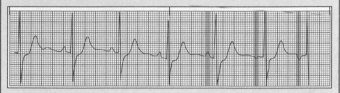

- Carefully examine the P waves. You'll be able to identify at least three different shapes of P waves (see shaded areas above) in a wandering pacemaker.
- Keep in mind that the atrial rhythm varies slightly, with an irregular P-P interval. The ventricular rhythm varies slightly as well, with an irregular R-R interval. These slight variations result from the changing site of impulse formation.

PACs

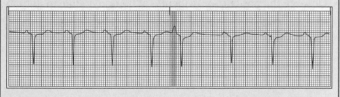

- Keep in mind that the PAC occurs earlier than the sinus P wave, with an abnormal configuration when compared with a sinus P wave (see shaded area above).
- It's possible, although rare, to see multifocal PACs that originate from multiple ectopic pacemaker sites in the atria. If this happens, the P waves may have different shapes.
- Except for the irregular atrial and ventricular rhythms that result from the PAC, the underlying rhythm is usually regular.

What causes it

- Increased parasympathetic (vagal) influences on the SA node or AV junction
- COPD
- Digoxin toxicity
- Inflammation of atrial tissue
- Valvular heart disease

What to look for

- Usually no symptoms (patient is unaware of the arrhythmia)
- Pulse rate normal or less than 60 beats/minute
- Rhythm regular or slightly irregular
- At least three distinct P-wave configurations (distinguish wandering pacemaker from PACs)

How it's treated

- Usually, no treatment is needed if the patient has no symptoms.
- If the patient has symptoms, his medication regimen should be reviewed and the underlying cause of the arrhythmia investigated and treated.
- Monitor the patient's heart rhythm.
- Observe the patient for evidence of hemodynamic instability, such as hypotension and changes in mental status.

Junctional arrhythmias

4

At this junction, we're going to discuss junctional arrhythmias. This type of arrhythmia occurs when impulses generate in the AV junction rather than the SA node.

Premature junctional contractions

- Also known as PJCs
- Junctional (ectopic) beats that occur before normal sinus beats and interrupt the underlying rhythm
- Impulses generated in the atrioventricular (AV) junction
- Commonly result from enhanced automaticity in junctional tissue or the bundle of His
- Retrograde depolarization of atria, causing an inverted P wave before, after, or hidden within the QRS complex
- Normal ventricular depolarization

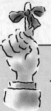

Memory jogger

To remember the location of the P wave in PJCs, recall that **A** comes *before* **V**, or **V** comes *after* **A**, in the term **AV junction:**

- If the atria (A) depolarize first, the P wave appears *before* the QRS complex.

- If the ventricles (V) depolarize first, the P wave appears *after* the QRS complex.

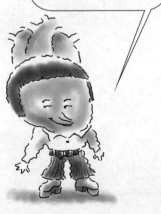

In premature junctional contractions, atrial depolarization occurs in a retro fashion. Groovy!

Recognizing PJCs

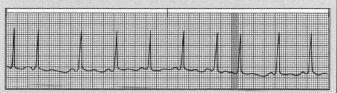

Rhythm
- Atrial: Irregular when PJCs occur
- Ventricular: Irregular when PJCs occur
- Underlying rhythm possibly regular

Rate
- Atrial: Reflects underlying rhythm
- Ventricular: Reflects underlying rhythm

P wave
- Usually inverted (leads II, III, and aV$_F$) or not visible
- May occur before, during, or after QRS complex, depending on initial direction of depolarization
- May be hidden in QRS complex

PR interval
- Shortened (less than 0.12 second) if P wave precedes QRS complex
- Not measurable if no P wave precedes QRS complex

QRS complex
- Usually normal configuration and duration because ventricles usually depolarize normally

T wave
- Usually normal configuration

QT interval
- Usually within normal limits

Other
- Commonly accompanied by a compensatory pause reflecting retrograde atrial conduction

What causes them

- Chronic obstructive pulmonary disease
- Coronary artery disease
- Digoxin toxicity
- Electrolyte imbalances
- Heart failure
- Hyperthyroidism
- Inferior-wall myocardial infarction (MI)

Locating the P wave

When specialized pacemaker cells in the AV junction take over as the dominant pacemaker of the heart, the P wave becomes inverted because the atria depolarize in a retrograde fashion. These illustrations show the various locations of P waves in junctional arrhythmias, depending on the depolarization sequence of the atria and ventricles.

If the atria depolarize first, the P wave will appear before the QRS complex.

Inverted P wave

If the ventricles depolarize first, the P wave will appear after the QRS complex.

Inverted P wave

If the ventricles and atria depolarize simultaneously, the P wave will be hidden in the QRS complex.

- Inflammatory changes in the AV junction after heart surgery
- Myocardial ischemia
- Pericarditis
- Stress
- Valvular heart disease

Triggers

- Alcohol
- Caffeine
- Nicotine

What to look for

- Usually no symptoms
- Possible feeling of palpitations or skipped beats
- Hypotension from a transient decrease in cardiac output if PJCs are frequent enough

How they're treated

- PJCs usually don't require treatment if the patient is asymptomatic.
- If the patient is symptomatic, the underlying cause should be treated.
- In patients taking digoxin, PJCs are a common early sign of toxicity. If the patient has digoxin toxicity, stop the drug and monitor the patient's drug levels as ordered.
- Monitor the patient's cardiac rhythm for frequent PJCs, which may indicate junctional irritability and can lead to a more serious arrhythmia such as junctional tachycardia.
- Monitor the patient for hemodynamic instability.
- If ectopic beats occur frequently because of a trigger such as caffeine intake, the patient should decrease or eliminate the trigger.

Junctional rhythm

- Also known as *junctional escape rhythm*
- Originates in the AV junction when the sinoatrial (SA) node fails as the dominant pacemaker, possibly for one of these reasons:
  – Firing rate of the SA node falls below the intrinsic firing rate of the AV junction
  – SA node fails to generate an impulse
  – Impulse conduction is blocked
- Atrial depolarization by retrograde conduction
- Normal conduction through ventricles
- Intrinsic firing rate for cells in AV junction: 40 to 60 beats/minute
- Protects the heart from potentially life-threatening idio-ventricular rhythms

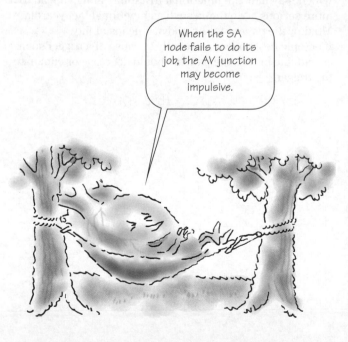

Recognizing junctional rhythm

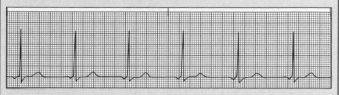

Rhythm
- Atrial: Regular
- Ventricular: Regular

Rate
- Atrial: 40 to 60 beats/minute
- Ventricular: 40 to 60 beats/minute

P wave
- Usually inverted (leads II, III, and aV$_F$)
- May occur before, during, or after QRS complex
- May be hidden in QRS complex

PR interval
- Shortened (less than 0.12 second) if P wave precedes QRS complex
- Not measurable if no P wave precedes QRS complex

QRS complex
- Duration: Usually within normal limits
- Configuration: Usually normal

T wave
- Configuration: Usually normal

QT interval
- Usually within normal limits

Other
- Important to differentiate junctional rhythm from idioventricular rhythm (a life-threatening arrhythmia)

What causes it

- Conditions that disturb normal SA node function or impulse conduction
- Cardiomyopathy
- Drugs
  - Beta-adrenergic blockers
  - Calcium channel blockers
  - Digoxin
- Electrolyte imbalances
- Heart failure
- Hypoxia

- Increased parasympathetic (vagal) tone
- Myocarditis
- SA node ischemia
- Sick sinus syndrome
- Valvular heart disease

Through the ages

Junctional rhythm: Age and life differences

Junctional escape beats may occur normally in healthy children during sleep. They may also occur in healthy athletic adults. In these situations, no treatment is necessary.

What to look for

- Possibly no symptoms
- Slow, regular pulse rate of 40 to 60 beats/minute (pulse rates below 60 beats/minute may lead to inadequate cardiac output, causing hypotension, syncope, or blurred vision)

How it's treated

- Because a junctional rhythm can prevent ventricular standstill, it should never be suppressed.
- Treatment for a junctional rhythm involves identification and correction of the underlying cause, whenever possible.
- Atropine or a transcutaneous, transvenous, or permanent pacemaker may be used to increase heart rate.
- Monitor the patient's digoxin and electrolyte levels.
- Watch for evidence of decreased cardiac output, such as hypotension, syncope, and blurred vision.

Junctional escape rhythm can help the heart escape a more dangerous condition.

Accelerated junctional rhythm

- Originates in the AV junction
- Involves enhanced automaticity of AV junctional tissue
- Occurs at 60 to 100 beats/minute (accelerated), exceeding the inherent junctional rate of 40 to 60 beats/minute
- Atrial depolarization by retrograde conduction
- Normal ventricular depolarization

Recognizing accelerated junctional rhythm

Rhythm
- Atrial: Regular
- Ventricular: Regular

Rate
- Atrial: 60 to 100 beats/minute
- Ventricular: 60 to 100 beats/minute

P wave
- If present, inverted in leads II, III, and aV$_F$
- May occur before, during, or after QRS complex
- May be hidden in QRS complex

PR interval
- Shortened (less than 0.12 second) if P wave precedes QRS complex

- Not measurable if no P wave precedes QRS complex

QRS complex
- Duration: Usually within normal limits but may be slightly prolonged
- Configuration: Usually normal

T wave
- Usually within normal limits

QT interval
- Usually within normal limits

Other
- Important to differentiate accelerated junctional rhythm from accelerated idioventricular rhythm (a possibly life-threatening arrhythmia)

What causes it
- Cardiac surgery
- Digoxin toxicity (common cause)
- Electrolyte disturbances
- Heart failure
- Inferior-wall MI
- Myocarditis
- Posterior-wall MI
- Rheumatic heart disease
- Valvular heart disease

What to look for
- Normal pulse rate and regular rhythm
- Possibly no symptoms because accelerated junctional rhythm has the same rate as sinus rhythm
- Possibly symptoms of decreased cardiac output (from loss of atrial kick), such as hypotension, changes in mental status, and weak peripheral pulses

How it's treated
- Treatment for accelerated junctional rhythm involves identifying and correcting the underlying cause.
- Assess the patient for signs and symptoms of decreased cardiac output and hemodynamic instability.
- Monitor the patient's serum digoxin and electrolyte levels.

Through the ages

Escape rate in young children
Up to age 3, the AV junctional escape rhythm is 50 to 80 beats/minute. Consequently, a junctional rhythm is considered accelerated in infants and toddlers only when it's greater than 80 beats/minute.

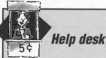

Help desk

Distinguishing accelerated junctional rhythm from accelerated idioventricular rhythm

An accelerated junctional rhythm and accelerated idioventricular rhythm appear similar but have different causes and require different interventions. To distinguish between them, closely examine the duration of the QRS complex and then look for P waves.

Accelerated junctional rhythm

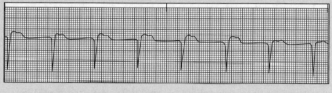

• The QRS complex duration and configuration are usually normal.
• Inverted P waves typically appear before or after the QRS complex, although P waves may be hidden in the QRS complex.
• The ventricular rate is usually 60 to 100 beats/minute.

Accelerated idioventricular rhythm

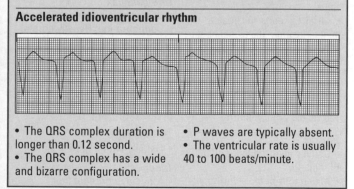

• The QRS complex duration is longer than 0.12 second.
• The QRS complex has a wide and bizarre configuration.
• P waves are typically absent.
• The ventricular rate is usually 40 to 100 beats/minute.

Junctional tachycardia

- Three or more PJCs in a row
- A supraventricular tachycardia
- Usually results from enhanced automaticity of the AV junction, which causes the AV junction to override the SA node as the dominant pacemaker

---

Recognizing junctional tachycardia

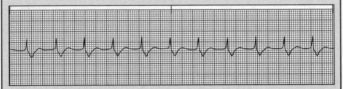

Rhythm
- Atrial: Usually regular but may be difficult to determine if P wave is hidden in QRS complex or preceding T wave
- Ventricular: Usually regular

Rate
- Atrial: Exceeds 100 beats/minute (usually 100 to 200 beats/minute) but may be difficult to determine if P wave is absent or hidden in QRS complex
- Ventricular: Exceeds 100 beats/minute (usually 100 to 200 beats/minute)

P wave
- Usually inverted in leads II, III, and aV$_F$
- May occur before, during, or after QRS complex
- May be hidden in QRS complex

PR interval
- Shortened (less than 0.12 second) if P wave precedes QRS complex
- Not measurable if no P wave precedes QRS complex

QRS complex
- Duration: Within normal limits
- Configuration: Usually normal

T wave
- Configuration: Usually normal
- May be abnormal if P wave is hidden in T wave
- May be indiscernible because of fast rate

QT interval
- Usually within normal limits

Other
- May have gradual (nonparoxysmal) or sudden (paroxysmal) onset

What causes it

- Digoxin toxicity (most common cause)
- Electrolyte imbalances
- Heart failure
- Hypokalemia (may aggravate condition)
- Inferior-wall MI
- Inferior-wall myocardial ischemia
- Inflammation of AV junction after heart surgery
- Posterior-wall MI
- Posterior-wall myocardial ischemia
- Valvular heart disease

What to look for

- Pulse rate above 100 beats/minute with a regular rhythm
- Effects of decreased cardiac output (loss of atrial kick) and hemodynamic instability (hypotension) in a patient with a rapid heart rate

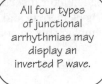

All four types of junctional arrhythmias may display an inverted P wave.

How it's treated

- The underlying cause should be identified and treated.
- If digoxin toxicity is the cause, digoxin should be discontinued. In some cases of digoxin toxicity, a digoxin-binding drug may be used to reduce serum digoxin levels.
- Vagal maneuvers and drugs such as adenosine may slow the heart rate for a symptomatic patient with paroxysmal onset of junctional tachycardia.

- If additional treatment is needed:
  - In patients with otherwise normal heart function, administer a beta-adrenergic blocker, calcium channel blocker, or amiodarone.
  - In patients with impaired heart function (heart failure or ejection fraction less than 40%), administer amiodarone.
- A patient with recurrent junctional tachycardia may be treated with ablation therapy followed by permanent pacemaker insertion.
- Check digoxin and potassium levels, and give potassium supplements as needed.

Ventricular arrhythmias

5

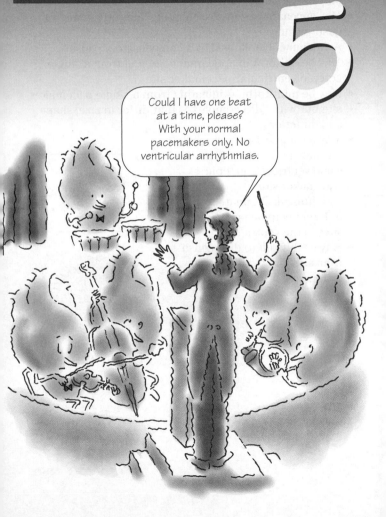

Premature ventricular contractions

- Also known as PVCs
- Ectopic beats that originate in the ventricles and occur earlier than expected
- May occur singly or in pairs (couplets), triplets, or clusters
- May appear in patterns, such as bigeminy, trigeminy, or quadrigeminy
- Are commonly followed by a compensatory pause
- May be uniform in appearance, arising from a single ectopic ventricular pacemaker site
- May be multiform, originating from a single pacemaker site but with QRS complexes that differ in size, shape, and direction
- May be unifocal or multifocal
  – Unifocal: Originate from the same ventricular ectopic pacemaker site
  – Multifocal: Originate from different ectopic pacemaker sites in the ventricles
- May be difficult to distinguish from aberrant ventricular conduction

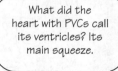

What did the heart with PVCs call its ventricles? Its main squeeze.

Recognizing PVCs

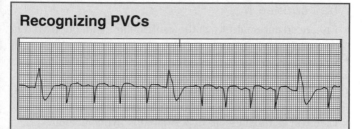

Rhythm
- Atrial: Irregular during PVCs
- Ventricular: Irregular during PVCs
- Underlying rhythm may be regular

Rate
- Atrial: Reflects underlying rhythm
- Ventricular: Reflects underlying rhythm

P wave
- Usually absent in ectopic beat
- May appear after QRS complex with retrograde conduction to atria
- Usually normal if present in underlying rhythm

PR interval
- Not measurable except in underlying rhythm

QRS complex
- Occurs earlier than expected
- Duration: Exceeds 0.12 second
- Configuration: Bizarre and wide but usually normal in underlying rhythm

T wave
- Opposite direction to QRS complex

- May trigger more serious rhythm disturbances when PVC occurs on the downslope of the preceding normal T wave (R-on-T phenomenon)

QT interval
- Not usually measured except in underlying rhythm

Other
- PVC may be followed by full or incomplete compensatory pause
- Full compensatory pause plus the preceding R-R interval equals the sum of two R-R intervals in underlying rhythm
- Incomplete compensatory pause plus the preceding R-R interval is less than the sum of two R-R intervals in underlying rhythm
- Interpolated PVC: Occurs between two normally conducted QRS complexes without great disturbance to underlying rhythm
- Full compensatory pause absent with interpolated PVCs
- May be difficult to distinguish PVCs from aberrant ventricular conduction

What causes it

- Enhanced automaticity in the ventricular conduction system or muscle tissue (usual cause)
- Irritable focus due to disruption of normal electrolyte shifts during cellular depolarization and repolarization
- Drug intoxication, particularly with amphetamines, cocaine, digoxin, phenothiazines, or tricyclic antidepressants
- Electrolyte imbalances (hyperkalemia, hypocalcemia, hypomagnesemia, hypokalemia)
- Enlargement of ventricular chambers
- Hypoxia
- Increased sympathetic stimulation
- Irritation of ventricles by pacemaker electrodes or a pulmonary artery catheter
- Metabolic acidosis
- Mitral valve prolapse
- Myocardial infarction (MI)
- Myocardial ischemia
- Myocarditis
- Sympathomimetic drugs, such as epinephrine and isoproterenol

Triggers

- Alcohol
- Caffeine
- Nicotine

What to look for

- Usually a normal pulse rate with a momentarily irregular pulse rhythm when a PVC occurs
- Possibly no symptoms
- Abnormally early heart sound with each PVC on auscultation
- Feeling of palpitations if PVCs are frequent
- Possible evidence of decreased cardiac output, including hypotension and syncope

Help desk

Distinguishing PVCs from ventricular aberrancy

PVCs and ventricular aberrancy are among the most challenging look-alike ECGs to distinguish. Sometimes they can be identified with complete confidence only in an electrophysiology lab.

Ventricular aberrancy, or aberrant ventricular conduction, occurs when an impulse originating in the sinoatrial (SA) node, atria, or atrioventricular (AV) junction is temporarily conducted abnormally through the bundle branches. This abnormal conduction results in bundle-branch block, usually because electrical impulses arrive at the bundle branches before the branches have been sufficiently repolarized.

To distinguish between PVCs and ventricular aberrancy, examine the deflection of the QRS complex in lead V_1. Then determine whether the QRS complex is primarily positive or negative. Based on this information, follow these clues to guide your analysis.

Mostly positive QRS complex
• Right bundle-branch aberrancy will have a triphasic rSR' configuration in V_1 and a triphasic qRS configuration in V_6.
• If there are two positive peaks in V_1 and the left peak is taller, the beat is probably a PVC.
• PVCs will be monophasic or biphasic in V_1, and biphasic in V_6, with a deep S wave.

PVC versus right bundle-branch aberrancy

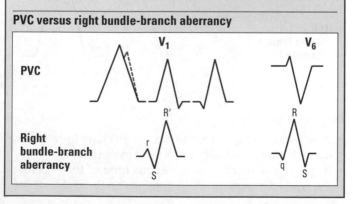

(continued)

Distinguishing PVCs from ventricular aberrancy *(continued)*

Mostly negative QRS complex
- Left bundle-branch aberrancy will have a narrow R wave with a quick downstroke in leads V_1 and V_2, and no Q wave in V_6.
- PVCs will have a wide R wave (greater than 0.03 second) and a notched or slurred S-wave downstroke in leads V_1 and V_2, with a duration greater than 0.06 second from the onset of the R wave to the deepest point of the S wave in V_1 and V_2, and a Q wave in V_6.
- P waves commonly precede aberrancies but typically don't precede PVCs.
- Aberrancies usually have a QRS duration of 0.12 second. PVCs are more likely to have a QRS duration of 0.14 second or more.

PVC versus left bundle-branch aberrancy

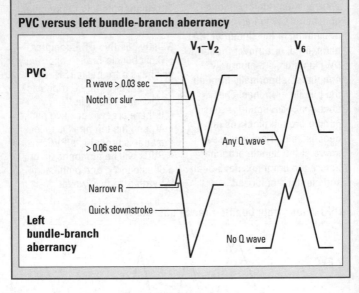

How it's treated
- If the patient is asymptomatic and doesn't have heart disease, the arrhythmia probably won't need to be treated.
- If symptoms occur, or a dangerous form of PVC occurs, the type of treatment given depends on the cause of the

problem. Symptoms may result from decreased cardiac output due to reduced ventricular diastolic filling time and loss of atrial kick.
- Until effective treatment begins, patients with PVCs and serious symptoms should have continuous ECG monitoring and should ambulate only with assistance.
- If PVCs are of a purely cardiac origin, drugs to suppress ventricular irritability may be used, such as:
  – amiodarone
  – lidocaine
  – procainamide.
- When PVCs have a noncardiac origin, treatment is aimed at correcting the cause. For example, treatment may include adjusting the patient's drug therapy or correcting acidosis.
- Patients who have recently developed PVCs need prompt assessment, especially if they have underlying heart disease or complex medical problems.
- Patients with chronic PVCs should be observed closely for the development of more frequent PVCs or more dangerous PVC patterns.
- If a patient is discharged with antiarrhythmic drugs, make sure that his family members know how to activate the emergency medical system and perform cardiopulmonary resuscitation (CPR).

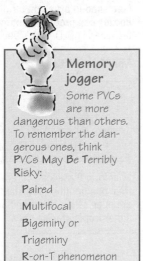

Memory jogger

Some PVCs are more dangerous than others. To remember the dangerous ones, think PVCs May Be Terribly Risky:

Paired

Multifocal

Bigeminy or

Trigeminy

R-on-T phenomenon

(Text continues on page 104.)

On the line

Patterns of potentially dangerous PVCs

Some PVCs are more dangerous than others. Here are some potentially dangerous ones.

Paired PVCs

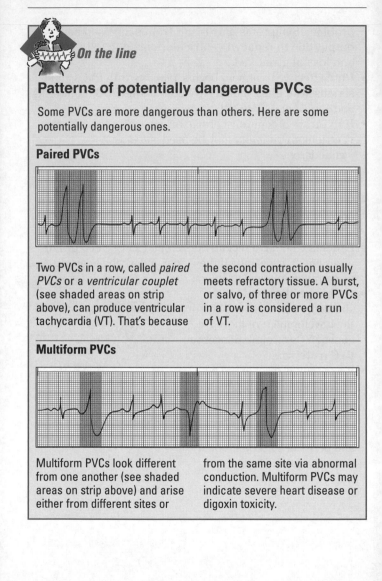

Two PVCs in a row, called *paired PVCs* or a *ventricular couplet* (see shaded areas on strip above), can produce ventricular tachycardia (VT). That's because the second contraction usually meets refractory tissue. A burst, or salvo, of three or more PVCs in a row is considered a run of VT.

Multiform PVCs

Multiform PVCs look different from one another (see shaded areas on strip above) and arise either from different sites or from the same site via abnormal conduction. Multiform PVCs may indicate severe heart disease or digoxin toxicity.

Patterns of potentially dangerous PVCs *(continued)*

Bigeminy and trigeminy

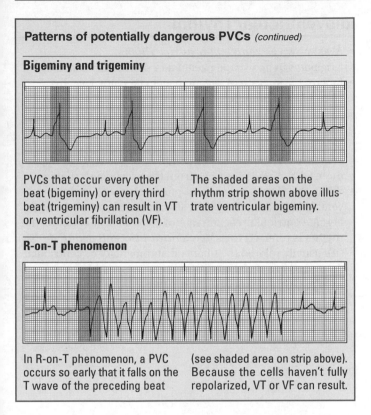

PVCs that occur every other beat (bigeminy) or every third beat (trigeminy) can result in VT or ventricular fibrillation (VF).

The shaded areas on the rhythm strip shown above illustrate ventricular bigeminy.

R-on-T phenomenon

In R-on-T phenomenon, a PVC occurs so early that it falls on the T wave of the preceding beat

(see shaded area on strip above). Because the cells haven't fully repolarized, VT or VF can result.

Idioventricular rhythm

- Also known as *ventricular escape rhythm*
- Originates in an escape pacemaker site in the ventricles
- Inherent firing rate of escape pacemaker site: Usually 20 to 40 beats/minute
- A safety mechanism because this rhythm prevents ventricular standstill (asystole [the absence of electrical activity in the ventricles])
- Ventricular escape beats or complexes: When fewer than three QRS complexes arise from the escape pacemaker
- When the rate of an ectopic pacemaker site in the ventricles is less than 100 beats/minute but exceeds the inherent ventricular escape rate of 20 to 40 beats/minute, the rhythm is referred to as *accelerated idioventricular rhythm* (it's usually related to enhanced automaticity of ventricular tissue and has the same ECG characteristics as idioventricular rhythm except for heart rate)

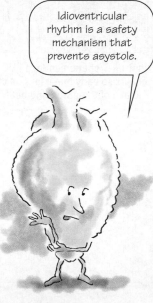

Idioventricular rhythm is a safety mechanism that prevents asystole.

On the line

Recognizing idioventricular rhythm

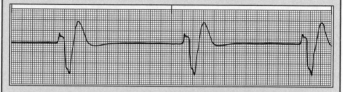

Rhythm
- Atrial: Usually can't be determined
- Ventricular: Usually regular

Rate
- Atrial: Usually can't be determined
- Ventricular: 20 to 40 beats/minute

P wave
- Usually absent

PR interval
- Not measurable because of absent P wave

QRS complex
- Duration: Exceeds 0.12 second because of abnormal ventricular depolarization
- Configuration: Wide and bizarre

T wave
- Abnormal
- Usually deflects in opposite direction from QRS complex

QT interval
- Usually prolonged

Other
- Commonly occurs with third-degree AV block
- If any P waves present, not associated with QRS complex

What causes it

- Digoxin toxicity
- Drugs
  - Beta-adrenergic blockers
  - Calcium channel blockers
  - Tricyclic antidepressants
- Failure of all of the heart's higher pacemakers
- Failure of supraventricular impulses to reach the ventricles because of a block in the conduction system

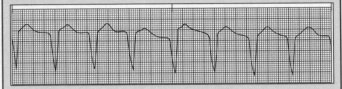

On the line

Recognizing accelerated idioventricular rhythm

Rhythm
- Atrial: Can't be determined
- Ventricular: Usually regular

Rate
- Atrial: Usually can't be determined
- Ventricular: 40 to 100 beats/minute

P wave
- Usually absent

PR interval
- Not measurable

QRS complex
- Duration: Exceeds 0.12 second
- Configuration: Wide and bizarre

T wave
- Abnormal
- Usually deflects in opposite direction from QRS complex

QT interval
- Usually prolonged

Other
- If any P waves present, not associated with QRS complex

- Metabolic imbalance
- MI
- Myocardial ischemia
- Pacemaker failure
- Sick sinus syndrome
- Third-degree heart block

What to look for

- Evidence of sharply decreased cardiac output (such as hypotension, dizziness, feeling of faintness, light-headedness, and syncope) if the patient has a continuous idioventricular rhythm
- Difficult auscultation or palpation of blood pressure

How it's treated

- Treatment should begin immediately to increase heart rate, improve cardiac output, and establish a normal rhythm.
- Treatment isn't intended to suppress the idioventricular rhythm because this arrhythmia acts as a safety mechanism against ventricular standstill.
- Never treat an idioventricular rhythm with antiarrhythmic drugs (such as amiodarone or lidocaine) because these drugs suppress the escape beats.
- Atropine may be given to increase heart rate. If atropine isn't effective or the patient develops hypotension or other evidence of clinical instability, a pacemaker may be inserted to reestablish a heart rate and cardiac output sufficient to perfuse organs.
- A transcutaneous pacemaker may be used in an emergency until a transvenous pacemaker can be inserted.
- Maintain continued ECG monitoring and periodically assess the patient until hemodynamic stability has been restored.
- Keep atropine and pacemaker equipment readily available.
- Enforce bed rest until an effective heart rate has been maintained and the patient is stable.
- Tell the patient and his family about the serious nature of this arrhythmia and the treatment it requires.
- If the patient needs a permanent pacemaker, explain how it works, how to recognize problems, when to contact a doctor, and how pacemaker function will be monitored.

Ventricular tachycardia

- Also called V-tach or VT
- Three or more PVCs in a row with a ventricular rate above 100 beats/minute
- May be monomorphic or polymorphic; sustained or non-sustained
- May progress quickly to VF and cardiovascular collapse because of decreased ventricular filling time and cardiac output
- May lead to torsades de pointes, a variation of polymorphic VT
- May be difficult to distinguish the relatively rare torsades de pointes from ventricular flutter
- May be difficult to distinguish VT from supraventricular tachycardia (SVT), especially if the patient has aberrant ventricular conduction

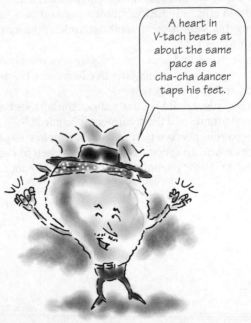

A heart in V-tach beats at about the same pace as a cha-cha dancer taps his feet.

On the line

Recognizing VT

Rhythm
• Atrial: Can't be determined
• Ventricular: Usually regular but may be slightly irregular

Rate
• Atrial: Can't be determined
• Ventricular: Usually rapid (100 to 250 beats/minute)

P wave
• Usually absent
• If present, not associated with QRS complex

PR interval
• Not measurable

QRS complex
• Duration: Exceeds 0.12 second
• Configuration: Usually bizarre, with increased amplitude

• Uniform in monomorphic VT
• Constantly changes shape in polymorphic VT

T wave
• If visible, occurs opposite the QRS complex

QT interval
• Not measurable

Other
• Ventricular flutter: A variation of VT
• Torsades de pointes: A variation of polymorphic VT that's relatively rare and sometimes difficult to distinguish from ventricular flutter

What causes it

• Usually increased myocardial irritability, which may be triggered by:
   – enhanced automaticity
   – PVCs during the downstroke of the preceding T wave
   – reentry in the Purkinje system

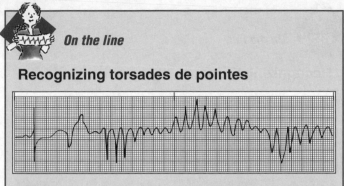

On the line

Recognizing torsades de pointes

Rhythm
- Atrial: Can't be determined
- Ventricular: May be regular or irregular

Rate
- Atrial: Can't be determined
- Ventricular: 150 to 300 beats/minute

P wave
- Not identifiable

PR interval
- Not measurable

QRS complex
- Usually wide
- Usually a phasic variation in electrical polarity, with complexes that point downward for several beats and then upward for several beats

T wave
- Not discernible

QT interval
- Prolonged

Other
- May be paroxysmal, starting and stopping suddenly

- Cardiomyopathy
- Coronary artery disease (CAD)
- Drug intoxication from cocaine, procainamide, or quinidine
- Electrolyte imbalances such as hypokalemia
- Heart failure
- Myocardial ischemia
- MI
- Rewarming during hypothermia
- Valvular heart disease

What to look for

- Possibly only minor symptoms initially
- Usually weak or absent pulses
- Hypotension and decreased level of consciousness due to decreased cardiac output, quickly leading to unresponsiveness if untreated
- Possible angina, heart failure, and substantial decrease in organ perfusion

How it's treated

- Determine whether the patient is conscious and has spontaneous respirations and a palpable carotid pulse.
- Patients with pulseless VT are treated the same as those with VF; they require immediate defibrillation.
- If the patient who has a pulse is unstable, perform immediate synchronized cardioversion.
- If the patient is stable, follow the monomorphic or polymorphic algorithm.
- A patient with chronic, recurrent episodes of VT who's unresponsive to drug therapy may need an implanted cardioverter-defibrillator (ICD).
- If a patient will be discharged with an ICD or on long-term antiarrhythmic therapy, make sure that family members know how to use the emergency medical system and how to perform CPR.

(Text continues on page 115.)

Through the ages

Pediatric torsades de pointes

Torsades de pointes at an early age is usually due to congenital long QT syndrome. Ask the parents about a family history of sudden cardiac death or sudden infant death syndrome.

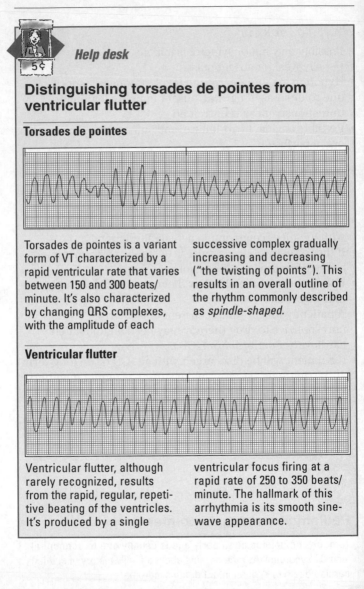

Help desk

Distinguishing torsades de pointes from ventricular flutter

Torsades de pointes

Torsades de pointes is a variant form of VT characterized by a rapid ventricular rate that varies between 150 and 300 beats/minute. It's also characterized by changing QRS complexes, with the amplitude of each successive complex gradually increasing and decreasing ("the twisting of points"). This results in an overall outline of the rhythm commonly described as *spindle-shaped.*

Ventricular flutter

Ventricular flutter, although rarely recognized, results from the rapid, regular, repetitive beating of the ventricles. It's produced by a single ventricular focus firing at a rapid rate of 250 to 350 beats/minute. The hallmark of this arrhythmia is its smooth sine-wave appearance.

Help desk

Distinguishing VT from SVT

Differentiating VT from SVT with aberrancy is difficult. However, careful assessment of a 12-lead ECG or rhythm strip can help you distinguish these arrhythmias with 90% accuracy. Begin by looking at the deflection — is it negative or positive? Then use the following illustrations to guide your assessment.

Negative deflection
If the QRS complex is wide and the deflection is mostly negative in lead V_1 or MCL_1, use these clues.

Ventricular tachycardia

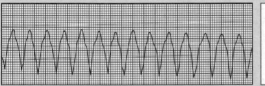 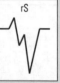

If the QRS complex has an R wave of 0.04 second or more, a slurred S (shown above, shaded), or a notched S on the downstroke (shown in inset above), suspect VT.

Supraventricular tachycardia

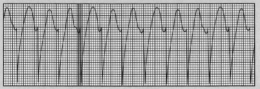 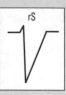

If the QRS complex has an R wave of 0.04 second or more and a swift, straight S on the downstroke (shown above, shaded, and in inset above), suspect SVT with aberrancy.

(continued)

Distinguishing VT from SVT *(continued)*

Positive deflection

If the QRS complex is wide and the deflection is mostly positive in lead V_1 or MCL_1, use these clues.

Ventricular tachycardia

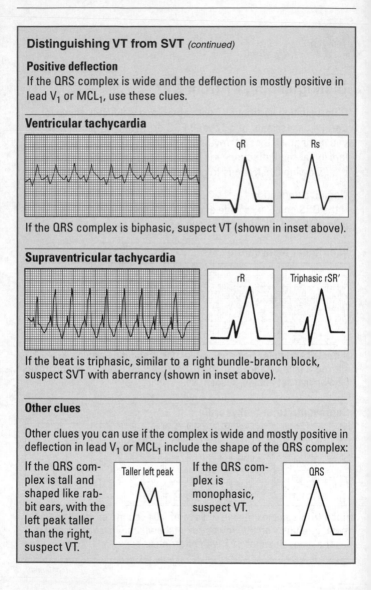

qR

Rs

If the QRS complex is biphasic, suspect VT (shown in inset above).

Supraventricular tachycardia

rR

Triphasic rSR′

If the beat is triphasic, similar to a right bundle-branch block, suspect SVT with aberrancy (shown in inset above).

Other clues

Other clues you can use if the complex is wide and mostly positive in deflection in lead V_1 or MCL_1 include the shape of the QRS complex:

If the QRS complex is tall and shaped like rabbit ears, with the left peak taller than the right, suspect VT.

Taller left peak

If the QRS complex is monophasic, suspect VT.

QRS

Distinguishing VT from SVT *(continued)*

If you still have trouble differentiating the rhythm, look at lead V_6 or MCL_6.

If the S wave is larger than the R wave, suspect VT.

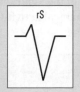

If a Q wave is present, suspect VT.

Additional criteria

Other criteria can also help you differentiate VT from SVT with aberrancy:

• A QRS complex that exceeds 0.14 second suggests VT.
• A regular, wide, complex rhythm suggests VT.
• An irregular, wide, complex rhythm suggests SVT with aberrancy.
• Concordant V leads (the QRS complex either mainly positive or mainly negative in all V leads) suggest VT.
• AV dissociation suggests VT.

• If a definitive diagnosis of SVT or VT can't be established, treatment should be guided by whether cardiac function is adequate (ejection fraction above 40%).
• Teach the patient and his family about the serious nature of this arrhythmia and the need for prompt treatment.

> A swift straight S on the downstroke suggests SVT with abberancy. Say that three times fast!

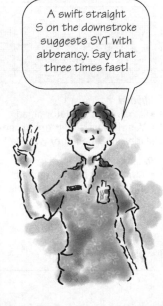

Ventricular fibrillation

- Commonly called V-fib or VF
- A chaotic, disorganized pattern of electrical impulses from multiple ectopic pacemakers in the ventricles
- No effective ventricular mechanical activity or contractions
- No cardiac output and no pulse

On the line

Recognizing VF

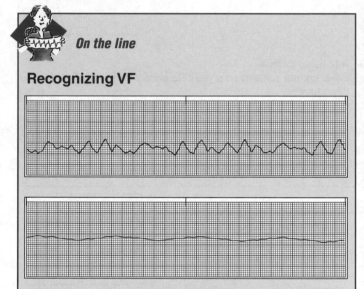

Rhythm
- Atrial: Can't be determined
- Ventricular: No pattern or regularity, just fibrillatory waves

Rate
- Atrial: Can't be determined
- Ventricular: Can't be determined

P wave
- Can't be determined

PR interval
- Can't be determined

QRS complex
- Can't be determined

T wave
- Can't be determined

QT interval
- Not applicable

Other
- Electrical defibrillation more successful with coarse fibrillatory waves than with fine waves

What causes it

- Acid-base imbalance
- CAD
- Drug toxicity, such as from digoxin, procainamide, or quinidine
- Electric shock
- Electrolyte imbalances, such as hypercalcemia, hyperkalemia, and hypokalemia
- MI
- Myocardial ischemia
- Severe hypothermia
- Underlying heart disease such as dilated cardiomyopathy
- Untreated VT

What to look for

- Full cardiac arrest
- Unresponsive patient with no detectable blood pressure or central pulses

How it's treated

- Start prompt treatment following health care facility and emergency medical system protocols.
- Assess the patient to determine if the rhythm is VF.
- Start CPR. To preserve the oxygen supply to the patient's brain and other vital organs, CPR must be performed until the defibrillator arrives and is fully charged.
- Defibrillate the patient immediately with 360 joules (monophasic defibrillator) or 120 to 200 joules (biphasic defibrillator).

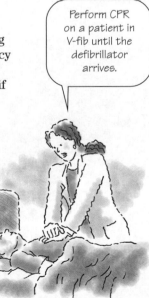

Perform CPR on a patient in V-fib until the defibrillator arrives.

- Administer epinephrine or vasopressin.
- Establish an airway and ventilate the patient.
- Consider giving an antiarrhythmic, such as amiodarone or lidocaine. Consider magnesium for torsades de pointes.
- Teach the patient and his family how to contact the emergency medical system and use an automated external defibrillator, if appropriate, after discharge from the facility.
- Instruct the patient's family how to perform CPR, if necessary.
- Teach the patient and his family about long-term therapies that help prevent recurrent episodes of VF, including anti-arrhythmic therapy and ICDs.

Asystole

- Also called *ventricular asystole* and *ventricular standstill*
- Characterized by absence of discernible electrical activity in the ventricles (possibly some electrical activity in the atria but no impulse conduction to the ventricles)
- Usually the result of prolonged cardiac arrest without effective resuscitation
- Important to distinguish from fine VF

On the line

Recognizing asystole

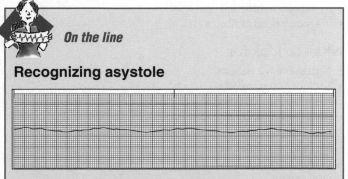

Rhythm
- Atrial: Usually indiscernible
- Ventricular: Not present

Rate
- Atrial: Usually indiscernible
- Ventricular: Not present

P wave
- May be present

PR interval
- Not measurable

QRS complex
- Absent or occasional escape beats

T wave
- Absent

QT interval
- Not measurable

Other
- Looks like a nearly flat line on a rhythm strip except during chest compressions with CPR
- If the patient has a pacemaker, pacer spikes may show on the strip, but no P wave or QRS complex occurs in response

What causes it

- Cardiac tamponade
- Drug overdose
- Hypothermia
- Hypovolemia
- Hypoxia
- Massive pulmonary embolism
- MI
- Severe electrolyte disturbances, especially hyperkalemia and hypokalemia
- Severe, uncorrected acid-base disturbances, especially metabolic acidosis
- Tension pneumothorax

What to look for

- Unresponsive patient
- Lack of spontaneous respirations, discernible pulse, and blood pressure
- No cardiac output or perfusion of vital organs

> Unlike with VT, a heart in asystole displays no rhythm on an ECG.

How it's treated

- Check to ensure that all electrodes are securely in place.
- Verify asystole by checking more than one ECG lead.
- Immediate treatment for asystole includes effective CPR, supplemental oxygen, and advanced airway control with tracheal intubation. (Resuscitation should be attempted unless evidence exists that it shouldn't be performed, such as when a do-not-resuscitate order is in effect.)
- Identify and treat potentially reversible causes; otherwise, asystole can quickly become irreversible.
- Give I.V. or intraosseous epinephrine and atropine. One dose of vasopressin may be given in place of the first or second dose of epinephrine.
- With hypothermia, rewarm the patient before making the decision to end resuscitation efforts.
- With persistent asystole despite appropriate management, resuscitation may end.

Pulseless electrical activity

- Also known as PEA
- Characterized by some electrical activity (may be any rhythm) but no mechanical activity or detectable pulse
- Electrical depolarization, but no synchronous shortening of myocardial fibers

On the line

Recognizing PEA

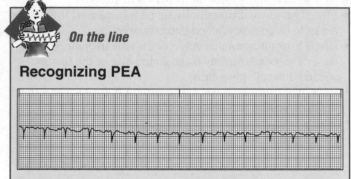

Rhythm
- Atrial: Same as underlying rhythm; becomes irregular as rate slows
- Ventricular: Same as underlying rhythm; becomes irregular as rate slows

Rate
- Atrial: Reflects underlying rhythm
- Ventricular: Reflects underlying rhythm; eventually decreases

P wave
- Same as underlying rhythm; gradually flattens and then disappears

PR interval
- Same as underlying rhythm; eventually disappears as P wave disappears

QRS complex
- Same as underlying rhythm; becomes progressively wider

T wave
- Same as underlying rhythm; eventually becomes indiscernible

QT interval
- Same as underlying rhythm; eventually becomes indiscernible

Other
- Usually becomes a flat line indicating asystole within several minutes

What causes it

- Acidosis
- Cardiac tamponade
- Hyperkalemia
- Hypokalemia
- Hypothermia
- Hypovolemia
- Hypoxia
- Massive acute MI or pulmonary embolism
- Overdoses of certain drugs such as tricyclic antidepressants
- Tension pneumothorax

What to look for

- Apnea and sudden loss of consciousness
- Lack of blood pressure and pulse and no cardiac output

How it's treated

- Start CPR immediately. Expect to give epinephrine and atropine according to advanced cardiac life support guidelines.
- Identify the cause of PEA and treat accordingly. Possible treatments include:
  - volume infusion for hypovolemia from hemorrhage
  - pericardiocentesis for cardiac tamponade
  - correction of electrolyte imbalances
  - needle decompression or chest tube insertion for tension pneumothorax
  - thrombolytic therapy for massive pulmonary embolism
  - ventilation for hypoxemia
  - rewarming for hypothermia.
- Pacemaker therapy isn't recommended.

Atrioventricular blocks

6

First-degree AV block

- Delay in conduction of electrical impulses through the normal conduction pathway
- Delayed at the level of the atrioventricular (AV) node or bundle of His
- Characterized by a PR interval that exceeds 0.20 second

Recognizing first-degree AV block

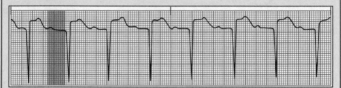

Rhythm
- Regular

Rate
- Within normal limits or brady-cardia
- Atrial the same as ventricular

P wave
- Normal size
- Normal configuration
- Each followed by a QRS complex

PR interval
- Prolonged
- More than 0.20 second (see shaded area on strip)
- Constant

QRS complex
- Within normal limits (0.08 second) if conduction delay occurs in AV node
- If more than 0.12 second, conduction delay may be in His-Purkinje system

T wave
- Normal size
- Normal configuration
- May be abnormal if QRS complex is prolonged

QT interval
- Within normal limits

What causes it

- Degenerative (age-related) changes in the heart
- Drugs
  - Beta-adrenergic blockers
  - Calcium channel blockers
  - Digoxin
  - Antiarrhythmics
- Myocardial infarction (MI)
- Myocardial ischemia
- Myocarditis

Through the ages

AV block in elderly patients

In elderly patients, AV block may be caused by conduction system fibrosis. Other causes include digoxin use and the presence of aortic valve calcification.

What to look for

- Normal or slow pulse rate
- Regular rhythm
- Usually no symptoms
- Usually no significant effect on cardiac output
- Increased interval between S_1 and S_2 heard on cardiac auscultation if the PR interval is extremely long

How it's treated

- Identify and correct the underlying cause.
- Monitor the patient's ECG to detect progression to a more serious block.

Type I second-degree AV block

- Also called *Wenckebach* or *Mobitz I block*
- Each impulse from the sinoatrial (SA) node is delayed slightly longer than previous impulse
- Pattern of progressive prolongation of PR interval
- Eventually, an impulse (usually a single impulse) isn't conducted to the ventricles
- Pattern repeated after nonconducted P wave or dropped beat

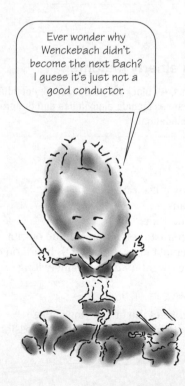

Ever wonder why Wenckebach didn't become the next Bach? I guess it's just not a good conductor.

Recognizing type I second-degree AV block

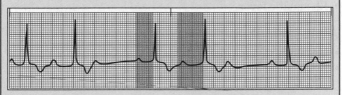

Rhythm
- Atrial: Regular
- Ventricular: Irregular

Rate
- Atrial rate exceeds ventricular rate because of non-conducted beats
- Both rates usually within normal limits

P wave
- Normal size
- Normal configuration
- Each followed by a QRS complex except blocked P wave

PR interval
- Progressively longer (see shaded areas on strip) with each cycle until a P wave appears without a QRS complex
- Commonly described as "long, longer, dropped"
- Slight variation in delay from cycle to cycle

- After the nonconducted beat, shorter than the interval preceding it

QRS complex
- Within normal limits (0.08 second)
- Periodically absent

T wave
- Normal size
- Normal configuration
- Deflection may be opposite that of the QRS complex

QT interval
- Usually within normal limits

Other
- Wenckebach pattern of grouped beats (footprints of Wenckebach)
- PR interval gets progressively longer and R-R interval shortens until a P wave appears without a QRS complex; cycle then repeats

What causes it

- Coronary artery disease (CAD)
- Drugs
  - Beta-adrenergic blockers
  - Digoxin
  - Calcium channel blockers

- Increased parasympathetic tone
- Inferior-wall MI
- Rheumatic fever

What to look for

- Usually no symptoms
- Evidence of decreased cardiac output
  - Hypotension
  - Syncope
- Pronounced signs and symptoms if ventricular rate is slow

How it's treated

- Monitor cardiac rhythm. The degree of the block may progress to a more serious form, especially if it occurs early in MI.
- Treat only symptomatic patients. This rhythm usually resolves when the underlying condition is corrected.
- Assess the patient's tolerance for the rhythm.
- Assess the need to improve cardiac output by observing for signs of decreased cardiac output, such as hypotension and syncope.
- Give atropine to improve AV node conduction.
- Use atropine cautiously if the patient is having an MI. Atropine can worsen ischemia.
- Maintain transcutaneous pacing, if needed, until the arrhythmia resolves.
- Teach the patient about a temporary pacemaker, if indicated.
- Evaluate the patient for possible causes (drugs, myocardial ischemia).
- Check the ECG for a more severe type of AV block.
- Ensure a patent I.V. line.

Type II second-degree AV block

- Also known as *Mobitz II block*
- Less common than type I but more serious
- Occasional failure of impulses from SA node to conduct to ventricles
- Occurs below level of AV node at bundle of His or bundle branches (more common)
- Hallmarks
  - Constant PR interval
  - Possibly more than one nonconducted beat in succession
- May be difficult to distinguish from nonconducted premature atrial contractions (PACs)

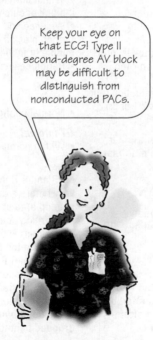

Keep your eye on that ECG! Type II second-degree AV block may be difficult to distinguish from nonconducted PACs.

(Text continues on page 133.)

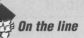

On the line

xtra "P"
Regular

Recognizing type II second-degree AV block

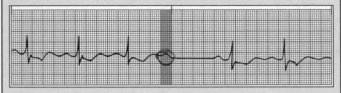

Rhythm
- Atrial: Regular
- Ventricular: Irregular
- Pauses correspond to dropped beat
- Irregular when block is intermittent or conduction ratio is variable
- Regular when conduction ratio is constant, such as 2:1 or 3:1

Rate
- Atrial exceeds ventricular
- Both may be within normal limits

P wave
- Normal size
- Normal configuration
- Some not followed by a QRS complex

PR interval
- Usually within normal limits but may be prolonged
- Constant for conducted beats
- May be shortened after a nonconducted beat

QRS complex
- Within normal limits or narrow if block occurs at bundle of His
- Widened and similar to bundle-branch block if block occurs at bundle branches
- Periodically absent

T wave
- Normal size
- Normal configuration

QT interval
- Within normal limits

Other
- PR and R-R intervals don't vary before a dropped beat (see shaded area on strip above), so no warning occurs
- R-R interval that contains nonconducted P wave equals two normal R-R intervals
- Must be a complete block in one bundle branch and intermittent interruption in conduction in the other bundle for a dropped beat to occur

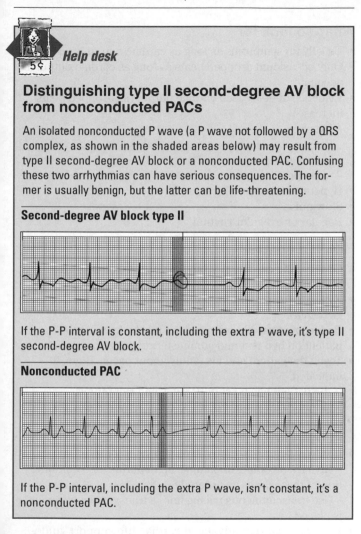

Help desk

Distinguishing type II second-degree AV block from nonconducted PACs

An isolated nonconducted P wave (a P wave not followed by a QRS complex, as shown in the shaded areas below) may result from type II second-degree AV block or a nonconducted PAC. Confusing these two arrhythmias can have serious consequences. The former is usually benign, but the latter can be life-threatening.

Second-degree AV block type II

If the P-P interval is constant, including the extra P wave, it's type II second-degree AV block.

Nonconducted PAC

If the P-P interval, including the extra P wave, isn't constant, it's a nonconducted PAC.

What causes it

- Anterior-wall MI
- Degenerative changes in the conduction system
- Severe CAD

What to look for

- Usually no symptoms as long as cardiac output is adequate
- Only occasional dropped beats as long as cardiac output is adequate
- Evidence of decreased cardiac output (as dropped beats increase)
  - Dyspnea
  - Fatigue
  - Light-headedness
  - Syncope
- Hypotension
- Slow pulse
- Regular or irregular rhythm

How it's treated

- Observe the cardiac rhythm for progression to a more severe block.
- Evaluate the patient for correctable causes (such as ischemia).
- Reduce myocardial oxygen demands by keeping the patient on bed rest and administering oxygen.
- Teach the patient and his family about pacemakers, if indicated.
- If the patient has no serious signs and symptoms:
  - Monitor him continuously, keeping a transcutaneous pacemaker attached to the patient or in the room.
  - Prepare him for transvenous pacemaker insertion.
- If the patient has serious signs and symptoms:
  - Give I.V. atropine, dopamine, epinephrine, or a combination of these drugs as ordered.
  - Use transcutaneous pacing until a transvenous pacemaker is placed.
- Keep in mind that advanced cardiac life support guidelines warn that atropine can worsen ischemia during an MI. It may induce ventricular tachycardia or fibrillation if the patient has Mobitz II block or complete heart block.

Third-degree AV block

- Also called *complete heart block*
- Complete absence of impulse conduction between the atria and ventricles
- Variable treatment and prognosis depending on anatomic level of block

At AV node, with a junctional escape rhythm

- Usually transient
- Usually favorable prognosis

At infranodal level

- Unstable pacemaker
- Common episodes of ventricular asystole
- Less-favorable prognosis
- Life-threatening because of slow ventricular rate and significantly decreased cardiac output

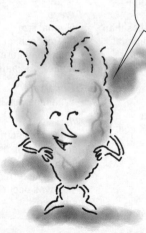

Third-degree AV block, you complete me. Completely block me, that is!

(Text continues on page 137.)

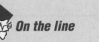

On the line

Recognizing third-degree AV block

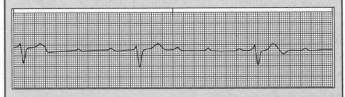

Rhythm
• Atrial: Regular
• Ventricular: Regular

Rate
• Atrial: 60 to 100 beats/minute (atria act independently under control of SA node)
• Ventricular: Usually 40 to 60 beats/minute in an intranodal block (a junctional escape rhythm)
• Ventricular: Usually less than 40 beats/minute in infranodal block (a ventricular escape rhythm)

P wave
• Normal size
• Normal configuration
• May be buried in QRS complex or T wave

PR interval
• Not measurable

QRS complex
• Configuration depends on location of escape mechanism and origin of ventricular depolarization
• Appears normal if the block is at the level of the AV node or bundle of His
• Widened if the block is at the level of the bundle branches

T wave
• Normal size
• Normal configuration
• May be abnormal if QRS complex originates in ventricle

QT interval
• Within normal limits

Other
• Atria and ventricles are depolarized from different pacemakers and beat independently of each other (AV dissociation)
• P waves occur without QRS complexes

What causes it

At level of AV node

- AV node damage
- Increased parasympathetic tone
- Inferior-wall MI
- Toxic effects of drugs (digoxin, propranolol)

At infranodal level

- Extensive anterior MI

Through the ages

Heart block after congenital heart repair

After repair of a ventricular septal defect, a child may require a permanent pacemaker if complete heart block develops. This arrhythmia may develop from interference with the bundle of His during surgery.

What to look for

- Possibly no symptoms except for exercise intolerance and unexplained fatigue
- Decreased cardiac output from loss of AV synchrony and resulting loss of atrial kick
- Changes in level of consciousness and mental status
- Chest pain
- Diaphoresis
- Dyspnea
- Hypotension
- Light-headedness
- Pallor
- Severe fatigue
- Slow peripheral pulse rate

How it's treated

- Make sure the patient has a patent I.V. line.
- Administer oxygen.
- Assess the patient for correctable causes of arrhythmia (drugs, myocardial ischemia).
- Minimize the patient's activity level.
- Restrict the patient to bed rest.
- If the patient has serious signs and symptoms, provide immediate treatment, including:
  – maintaining transcutaneous pacing (most effective)
  – giving I.V. dopamine, epinephrine, or a combination (for short-term use in emergencies).
- Keep in mind that atropine isn't indicated for third-degree AV block, especially when accompanied by wide-complex ventricular escape beats.
- If the patient has symptoms, maintain temporary transvenous pacing until the need for a permanent pacemaker is determined.

ECG effects of electrolyte imbalances

7

Electrolyte imbalances can really throw me off kilter. Read this chapter to find out what that looks like on an ECG.

Hyperkalemia

- Serum potassium level above 5 mEq/L

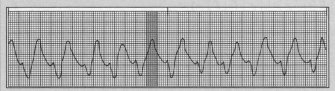

ECG effects of hyperkalemia

Rhythm
- Regular

Rate
- Within normal limits

P wave
- Low amplitude in mild hyperkalemia
- Wide and flattened in moderate hyperkalemia
- Not discernible in severe hyperkalemia

PR interval
- Normal or prolonged
- Not measurable if P wave can't be detected

QRS complex
- Widened

T wave
- Tall and peaked (the key finding, as shown in shaded area on strip)

QT interval
- Shortened

Other
- Intraventricular conduction disturbances are common
- ST segment may be elevated in severe hyperkalemia

What causes it

- Increased potassium intake via:
  - diet, including salt substitutes
  - I.V. administration of penicillin G, potassium supplements, or banked whole blood

- A shift of potassium from intracellular to extracellular fluid with changes in cell membrane permeability or damage caused by:
  – acidosis
  – burns
  – cell hypoxia
  – extensive surgery
  – insulin deficiency
  – massive crush injuries
- Decreased renal excretion caused by:
  – Addison's disease
  – decreased production and secretion of aldosterone
  – renal failure
  – use of potassium-sparing diuretics

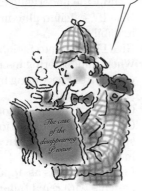

I think I've got it! P waves shrink or disappear as potassium levels rise.

What to look for

Mild hyperkalemia

- Diarrhea
- Intestinal cramping
- Neuromuscular irritability
- Restlessness
- Tingling lips and fingers

Severe hyperkalemia

- Loss of muscle tone
- Ascending skeletal muscle weakness
- Flaccid paralysis
- Cardiac arrhythmias

How it's treated

- Appropriate interventions vary according to:
  - severity of hyperkalemia
  - patient's signs and symptoms.
- Identify the underlying cause.
- Give I.V. calcium gluconate to decrease neuromuscular irritability.
- Give I.V. insulin to facilitate entry of potassium into cells.
- When administering insulin to treat hyperkalemia, keep the patient from becoming hypoglycemic by giving I.V. dextrose at the same time.
- Give I.V. sodium bicarbonate to correct metabolic acidosis.
- Give oral or rectal cation exchange resins (sodium polystyrene sulfonate) that exchange sodium for potassium in the intestine.
- Perform dialysis as appropriate. Dialysis may be used in patients with renal failure or severe hyperkalemia to remove excess potassium.
- Monitor serum potassium levels closely.
- Identify and manage arrhythmias.

Hypokalemia

- Potassium level below 3.5 mEq/L

ECG effects of hypokalemia

Rhythm
- Regular

Rate
- Within normal limits

P wave
- Normal size
- Normal configuration
- May be peaked in severe hypokalemia

PR interval
- May be prolonged

QRS complex
- Within normal limits
- Possibly widened
- Prolonged in severe hypokalemia

T wave
- Has decreased amplitude
- Becomes flat as potassium level drops, and U wave appears (the key finding, as shown in shaded area on strip)
- Flattens completely in severe hypokalemia and may become inverted
- May fuse with increasingly prominent U wave

QT interval
- Usually indiscernible as T wave flattens

Other
- Depressed ST segment
- Increased amplitude and prominence of U wave as hypokalemia worsens; may fuse with T wave

What causes it

- Potassium loss through abnormal routes
  - Continuous nasogastric drainage
  - Diarrhea

  - Drainage tubes
  - Intestinal fistulae
  - Laxative abuse
  - Vomiting
- Increased secretion of potassium by the distal tubule
- Low serum magnesium level
- Excessive aldosterone secretion
- Drugs
  - Antibiotics, such as amphotericin B or gentamicin
  - Diuretics
  - Corticosteroids
- Increased entry of potassium into cells due to alkalosis, especially respiratory
- Reduced potassium intake or dietary deficiency due to anorexia or nothing-by-mouth status

What to look for

- Signs and symptoms of smooth-muscle atony
  - Anorexia
  - Constipation
  - Intestinal distention
  - Paralytic ileus
  - Nausea
  - Vomiting
- Skeletal muscle weakness (first appearing in larger muscles of the arms and legs and eventually in the diaphragm, causing respiratory arrest)
- Cardiac arrhythmias
  - Atrioventricular block
  - Bradycardia
  - Ventricular arrhythmias

How it's treated

- Identify and correct the underlying cause.
- Correct acid-base imbalances.
- Replace potassium losses and prevent further losses.

- Encourage intake of potassium-rich foods and fluids.
- Give oral or I.V. potassium supplements.
- Monitor serum potassium levels closely.
- Keep in mind that hypokalemia may result in digoxin toxicity. Monitor serum digoxin and potassium levels closely at the start of therapy and until maintenance doses are determined.
- Identify and manage cardiac arrhythmias.
- Monitor the patient closely for early evidence of skeletal muscle weakness because it may progress to respiratory arrest.

Hypercalcemia

- Serum calcium level above 10.5 mg/dl

ECG effects of hypercalcemia

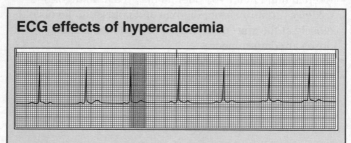

Rhythm
- Regular

Rate
- Within normal limits
- Possible bradycardia

P wave
- Normal size
- Normal configuration

PR interval
- May be prolonged

QRS complex
- Within normal limits
- May be prolonged

T wave
- Normal size
- Normal configuration
- May be depressed

QT interval
- Shortened from increased calcium level (the key finding, as shown in shaded area on strip)

Other
- Shortened ST segment

What causes it

- Conditions that shift calcium from bone into extracellular fluid
  - Bone metastasis and calcium resorption from cancers of the breast, prostate, or cervix
  - Hyperparathyroidism
  - Parathyroid hormone (PTH)–producing tumors
  - Sarcoidosis
- Increased calcium intake or absorption

- Excess vitamin D intake
- Decreased calcium excretion (possibly caused by thiazide diuretics)

What to look for
- Anorexia
- Behavior changes
- Constipation
- Fatigue
- Impaired renal function
- Lethargy
- Nausea or vomiting
- Reciprocal decrease in serum phosphate levels
- Renal calculi (precipitates of calcium salts)
- Muscle weakness
- Slurred speech

How it's treated
- Identify and manage the underlying cause.
- Use the severity of the patient's symptoms to guide treatment.
- If renal function is normal, give oral phosphates.
- Administer large volumes of I.V. normal saline solution to enhance renal excretion of calcium.
- Give corticosteroids and calcitonin.
- Patients with renal failure receive dialysis.

I don't want to sound hyper, but too much calcium can be problematic.

Hypocalcemia

- Serum calcium level below 8.5 mg/dl.

ECG effects of hypocalcemia

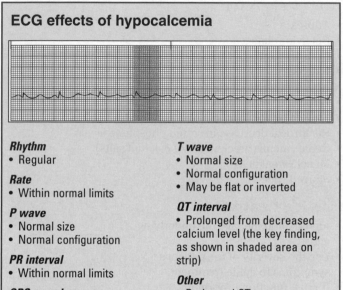

Rhythm
- Regular

Rate
- Within normal limits

P wave
- Normal size
- Normal configuration

PR interval
- Within normal limits

QRS complex
- Within normal limits

T wave
- Normal size
- Normal configuration
- May be flat or inverted

QT interval
- Prolonged from decreased calcium level (the key finding, as shown in shaded area on strip)

Other
- Prolonged ST segment

What causes it

- Inadequate calcium intake due to diet deficient in green, leafy vegetables and dairy products
- Excessive phosphorus intake (binds with calcium and prevents calcium absorption)
- Pancreatitis (decreases ionized calcium)
- Blood administration (the citrate solution in stored blood binds with calcium)
- Neoplastic bone metastasis (decrease serum calcium levels)
- Vitamin D deficiency due to inadequate intake or inadequate exposure to sunlight

- Malabsorption of fats
- Inadequate PTH levels (caused by removal of parathyroid glands)
- Metabolic or respiratory alkalosis
- Hypoalbuminemia (low albumin level)

What to look for

- Carpopedal spasm
- Circumoral or digital paresthesia
- Confusion
- Hyperactive bowel sounds
- Hyperreflexia
- Intestinal cramping
- Positive Chvostek's sign
- Positive Trousseau's sign

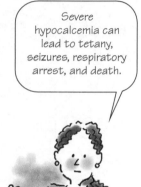

Severe hypocalcemia can lead to tetany, seizures, respiratory arrest, and death.

Severe hypocalcemia

- Tetany
- Seizures
- Respiratory arrest
- Death

How it's treated

- Identify and manage the underlying cause.
- Monitor serum calcium levels.
- Administer I.V. calcium gluconate for severe symptoms. Keep calcium gluconate on hand for a patient with a positive Trousseau's or Chvostek's sign. Hypocalcemia may progress quickly to tetany, seizures, respiratory arrest, and death.
- Replace calcium orally.
- Identify and manage cardiac arrhythmias.
- Instruct the patient to decrease phosphate intake.

ECG effects of antiarrhythmics

8

Class I antiarrhythmics

- Also known as *sodium channel blockers* or *fast channel blockers*
- Block sodium influx during phase 0 of action potential
- Subdivided into three groups (classes IA, IB, and IC) based on drug effects
  - Interference with cardiac sodium channel function
  - Effects on duration of action potential

Class IA antiarrhythmics

- Examples
  - Disopyramide
  - Procainamide
  - Quinidine
- Have intermediate interaction with sodium channels
- Cardiac effects
  - Lengthen duration of action potential
  - Depress rate of depolarization
  - Prolong repolarization
  - Lengthen refractory period
  - Reduce conductivity
  - Decrease automaticity

Talk about potential! The four classes of antiarrhythmics each affect a different segment of the action potential.

ECG effects of class IA antiarrhythmics

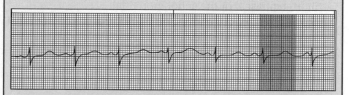

Rhythm
- No change in underlying rhythm

Rate
- No change

P wave
- No change

PR interval
- No change

QRS complex
- Slightly widened

- Increased widening: An early sign of toxicity

T wave
- Possibly flattened or inverted

QT interval
- Prolonged (see shaded area on strip), increases the probability of polymorphic ventricular tachycardia

Other
- Possible U wave

Class IB antiarrhythmics

- Examples
  - Lidocaine
  - Mexiletine
  - Phenytoin
  - Tocainide
- Interact rapidly with sodium channels
- May block sodium influx during phase 0, which depresses rate of depolarization

Think of antiarrhythmics as cardiac linebackers. They block sodium (class I), beta receptors (II), potassium (III), and calcium (IV). Go team!

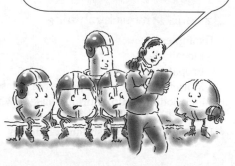

- Cardiac effects
  - Slow phase 0 of the action potential
  - Shorten phase 3 of the action potential
  - May shorten repolarization and duration of action potential
  - Suppress ventricular ectopy
  - May suppress ventricular automaticity in ischemic tissue
  - May widen QRS complex

ECG effects of class IB antiarrhythmics

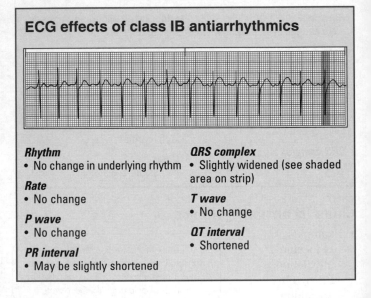

Rhythm
- No change in underlying rhythm

Rate
- No change

P wave
- No change

PR interval
- May be slightly shortened

QRS complex
- Slightly widened (see shaded area on strip)

T wave
- No change

QT interval
- Shortened

Class IC antiarrhythmics

- Examples
  - Flecainide
  - Propafenone
  - Moricizine (shares properties of classes IA, IB, and IC)
- Block sodium influx during phase 0, which depresses the rate of depolarization
- Interact slowly with sodium channels

- Cardiac effects
  – May have no effect on action potential duration or may minimally increase it
  – Slow phase 0 of action potential
  – Decrease conduction
  – Don't affect repolarization
- Are usually reserved for refractory arrhythmias because they may cause or worsen arrhythmias

ECG effects of class IC antiarrhythmics

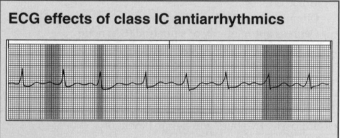

Rhythm
- No change in underlying rhythm

Rate
- No change

P wave
- No change

PR interval
- Prolonged (see shaded area above left)

QRS complex
- Widened (see middle shaded area)

T wave
- No change

QT interval
- Prolonged (see shaded area above right)

Class II antiarrhythmics

- Also known as *beta-adrenergic blockers*
- Examples
  - Acebutolol
  - Esmolol
  - Propranolol
- Block beta receptors in sympathetic nervous system
- Inhibit sympathetic stimulation
- Cardiac effects
  - Diminish phase 4 depolarization
  - Depress automaticity of sinoatrial (SA) node
  - Increase refractory period of atrial and atrioventricular (AV) junctional tissues, which slows conduction
  - Decrease myocardial oxygen demand
- Used to treat supraventricular and ventricular arrhythmias, especially those caused by excess circulating catecholamines
- Cardioselective beta-adrenergic blockers
  - Block only beta$_1$ receptors
- Noncardioselective beta-adrenergic blockers
  - May block beta$_1$ and beta$_2$ receptors
  - May cause vasoconstriction
  - May cause bronchospasm
- Should be used cautiously in patients with pulmonary disease because it may cause bronchial constriction
- Can mask signs and symptoms of hypoglycemia

ECG effects of class II antiarrhythmics

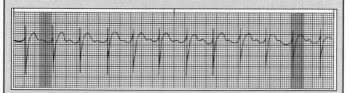

Rhythm
• No change in underlying rhythm

Rate
• Atrial: Decreased
• Ventricular: Decreased

P wave
• No change

PR interval
• Slightly prolonged (see shaded area above left)

QRS complex
• No change

T wave
• No change

QT interval
• Slightly shortened (see shaded area above right)

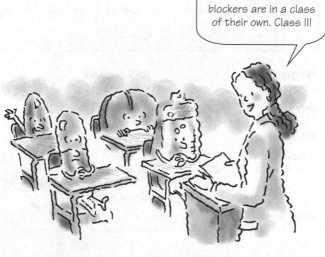

Class III antiarrhythmics

- Also known as *potassium channel blockers*
- Block movement of potassium during phase 3 of the action potential
- Examples
  - Amiodarone
  - Dofetilide
  - Ibutilide
  - Sotalol (a nonselective beta-adrenergic blocker with mainly class III properties)
- Cardiac effects
  - Increase duration of action potential and effective refractory period
  - Prolong repolarization

ECG effects of class III antiarrhythmics

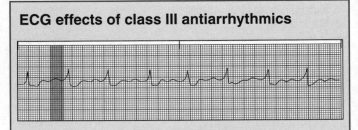

Rhythm
- No change

Rate
- No change or possibly decreased

P wave
- No change

PR interval
- Prolonged (see shaded area above left)

QRS complex
- Widened (see middle shaded area)

T wave
- No change or decreased amplitude

QT interval
- Prolonged (see shaded area above right)

Class IV antiarrhythmics

- Also known as *calcium channel blockers* or *slow channel blockers*
- Block movement of calcium during phase 2 of the action potential
- Examples
  - Diltiazem
  - Verapamil

Through the ages

Prolonged diltiazem effects in elderly patients

Administer diltiazem cautiously to an older adult because the half-life of the drug may be prolonged. Be especially careful if the older adult also has heart failure or impaired hepatic or renal function.

- Cardiac effects
  - Slow conduction
  - Increase refractory period of calcium-dependent tissues, including the AV node
  - Decrease contractility

ECG effects of class IV antiarrhythmics

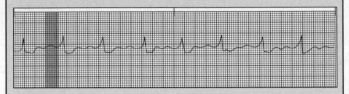

Rhythm
- No change

Rate
- Atrial: Decreased
- Ventricular: Decreased

P wave
- No change

PR interval
- Prolonged (see shaded area on strip)

QRS complex
- No change

T wave
- No change

QT interval
- No change

Digoxin

- Most commonly used cardiac glycoside
- Inhibits adenosine triphosphatase, an enzyme found in the plasma membrane that:
  - acts as a pump to exchange sodium ions for potassium ions
  - enhances movement of calcium from extracellular space to intracellular space
  - strengthens myocardial contractions
- Exerts direct effects on electrical properties of the heart
  - Shortens action potential
  - May shorten atrial and ventricular refractory period
- Exerts autonomic effects on electrical properties of the heart
  - Involves parasympathetic system
  - Enhances vagal tone
  - Slows conduction through the SA and AV nodes
- Is used to treat heart failure
- Is used to treat certain arrhythmias
  - Paroxysmal supraventricular tachycardia
  - Atrial fibrillation (to slow ventricular response rate)
  - Atrial flutter (to slow ventricular response rate)
- Has a very narrow range of therapeutic effectiveness
- May produce toxic levels
- At toxic levels, may cause numerous arrhythmias, including paroxysmal atrial tachycardia with block, AV block, atrial and junctional tachyarrhythmias, and ventricular arrhythmias.

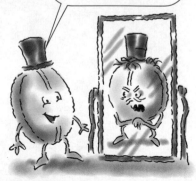

You've gotta watch out for my dark side. Although I can be used to treat arrhythmias, at toxic levels, I can also cause them.

ECG effects of digoxin

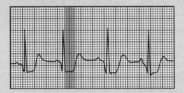

Rhythm
• No change

Rate
• Atrial: Decreased
• Ventricular: Decreased

P wave
• Possibly notched

PR interval
• Shortened

QRS complex
• No change

T wave
• Decreased amplitude

QT interval
• Shortened because of shortened ST segment

Other
• Characteristic sagging (scooping or sloping) of ST segment
• ST segment depressed in opposite direction of QRS deflection (see shaded area on strip)
• Shortened ST segment

Pacemakers and ICDs

9

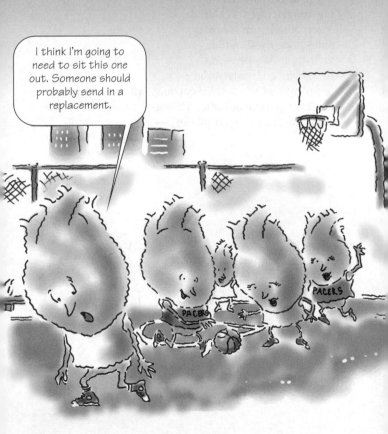

Pacemaker basics

- A pacemaker is a device that stimulates depolarization of the myocardium by generating electrical impulses and conducting them to the heart.
- Pacemakers are typically needed after myocardial infarction (MI) or cardiac surgery.
- Pacemakers are commonly used to treat irreversible heart conduction problems.
- They're also indicated for:
  - atrioventricular (AV) block
  - symptomatic bradycardia
  - sinus node dysfunction
  - arrhythmia suppression
  - drug-induced bradycardia
  - improvement of exercise capacity with rate response
  - cardiac resynchronization (biventricular pacing for heart failure).

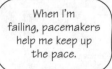

When I'm failing, pacemakers help me keep up the pace.

Pacemaker components

- Pacemakers have three main components:
  - pulse generator
  - pacing leads or wires
  - one or more electrodes at the distal ends of the leadwires.

Pulse generator

- The generator contains a power source (battery) and electronic circuitry.
- It creates an electrical impulse that moves through the pacing leads to the electrodes, which transmit that impulse to the heart muscle, causing the heart to depolarize.
- The batteries typically contain lithium iodide and can last 5 to 10 years depending on the frequency of pacing.
- Sensing, output, and timing circuits determine how the pacemaker responds to the heart's electrical activity.
- A microprocessor (computer chip with memory) can increase the pacemaker's capabilities and data storage.
- Telemetry can be used to allow communication between the pulse generator and an external programmer for reprogramming and data retrieval.

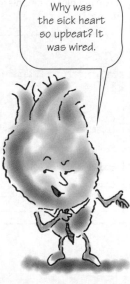

Why was the sick heart so upbeat? It was wired.

Leads and electrodes

- Leads consist of insulated conductors (low-voltage wires) and electrodes.
- Electrodes sense the heart's electrical activity.
- Leads carry information from the electrodes to the pulse generator and electrical impulses from the generator to the heart muscle.

- In single-chamber pacing, a lead is placed in the right atrium or right ventricle.
- In dual-chamber or AV pacing, leads are placed in both the right atrium and right ventricle.
- In biventricular pacing, leads are placed in the right atrium, right ventricle, and coronary sinus.
- Pacing leads have either one electrode (unipolar) or two (bipolar).

Pacing leads

Unipolar lead

In a unipolar (one lead) system, electrical current moves from the pulse generator through the leadwire to the negative pole. From there, it stimulates the heart and returns to the pulse generator's metal surface (the positive pole) to complete the circuit.

Bipolar lead

In a bipolar (two lead) system, current flows from the pulse generator through the leadwire to the negative pole at the tip. At that point, it stimulates the heart and then flows back to the positive pole to complete the circuit.

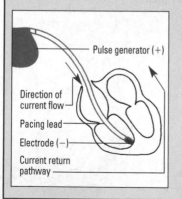

Pulse generator (+)
Direction of current flow
Pacing lead
Electrode (−)
Current return pathway

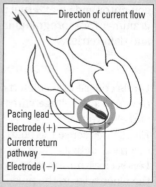

Direction of current flow
Pacing lead
Electrode (+)
Current return pathway
Electrode (−)

ECG effects of pacemakers

- The most notable ECG characteristic produced by a pacemaker is known as a *pacemaker spike*.
- A pacemaker spike:
  - occurs when the pacemaker sends an electrical impulse to the heart muscle
  - appears as a vertical line on the ECG tracing
  - is usually small and can be difficult to see in certain leads.

When the pacemaker stimulates the atria

- The spike is followed by a P wave.
- This pattern represents successful pacing (known as *capture*) of the atrial myocardium.
- The P wave may appear different from the patient's normal P wave.

When the pacemaker stimulates the ventricles

- The spike is followed by a QRS complex and a T wave.
- This pattern represents successful pacing (capture) of the ventricular myocardium.
- The QRS complex appears wider than the patient's own QRS complex because of the way the pacemaker depolarizes the ventricles.

When the pacemaker stimulates both the atria and ventricles

- The atrial spike is followed by a P wave, and then a ventricular spike, and then a QRS complex.
- This pattern represents successful pacing (capture) of the atrial and ventricular myocardium.

Pacemaker spikes

Pacemaker impulses — the stimuli that travel from the pacemaker to the heart — appear as spikes on an ECG tracing. Whether large or small, pacemaker spikes appear above or below the isoelectric line. The illustration below shows an atrial pacemaker spike and a ventricular pacemaker spike.

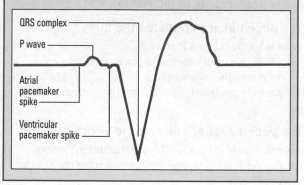

Pacemaker programming

Synchronous and asynchronous pacemakers

- Pacemakers are classified as synchronous or asynchronous according to how they stimulate the heart:
  – A synchronous, or demand, pacemaker responds to the heart's activity by monitoring the intrinsic rhythm and pacing only when the heart can't do so itself.
  – An asynchronous, or fixed-rate, pacemaker fires at a preset heart rate regardless of the heart's intrinsic cycle. This type of pacemaker is rarely used.

Pacemaker codes

- A code, usually three or four letters long, is commonly used to describe pacemaker mode or function.

Pacing modes

- *Pacing mode* refers to the programming and capabilities of a particular device.
- A mode is selected based on the status of the patient's intrinsic heart rhythm and the indication for pacing.

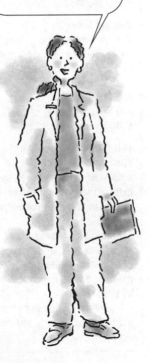

The pacing mode depends mostly on the chamber of the heart that the pacemaker senses and paces.

(Text continues on page 173.)

Pacemaker coding systems

The capabilities of permanent pacemakers can be described by a five-letter coding system. Typically, only the first three letters are used.

First letter
The first letter identifies which heart chambers are paced:
- V = Ventricle
- A = Atrium
- D = Dual — ventricle and atrium
- O = None

Second letter
The second letter signifies the heart chamber where the pacemaker senses intrinsic activity:
- V = Ventricle
- A = Atrium
- D = Dual
- O = None

Third letter
The third letter indicates the pacemaker's mode of response to the intrinsic electrical activity it senses in the atrium or ventricle:
- T = Triggers pacing
- I = Inhibits pacing
- D = Dual — can be triggered or inhibited depending on the mode and where intrinsic activity occurs
- O = None — doesn't change mode in response to sensed activity

Fourth letter
The fourth letter describes the degree of programmability and the presence or absence of an adaptive rate response:
- P = Basic functions programmable
- M = Multiprogrammable parameters
- C = Communicating functions, such as telemetry
- R = Rate responsiveness — rate adjusts to fit the patient's metabolic needs and achieve normal hemodynamic status
- O = None

Fifth letter
The fifth letter denotes the pacemaker's response to a tachyarrhythmia:
- P = Pacing ability — the pacemaker's rapid burst paces the heart at a rate above its intrinsic rate to override the tachycardia source
- S = Shock — an ICD identifies ventricular tachycardia and delivers a shock to stop the arrhythmia
- D = Dual ability to shock and pace
- O = None

AAI and VVI pacemakers

AAI and VVI pacemakers are single-chamber pacemakers. The electrode is placed in the atrium for an AAI pacemaker and in the ventricle for a VVI pacemaker. These rhythm strips show how each pacemaker works.

AAI pacemaker

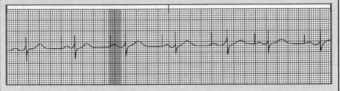

An AAI pacemaker senses and paces only the atria. As shown in the shaded area above, a P wave follows each atrial spike (atrial depolarization). The QRS complexes reflect the heart's own conduction.

This type of pacemaker requires a functioning AV node and intact conduction system. It may be used in patients who have symptomatic sinus brady-cardia or sick sinus syndrome.

VVI pacemaker

A VVI pacemaker senses and paces the ventricles. When each spike is followed by a QRS complex (depolarization), as shown in the shaded area above, the rhythm is said to reflect 100% capture.

This pacemaker may be used in patients who have chronic atrial fibrillation with slow ven-tricular response or those who need infrequent pacing.

DDD pacemaker

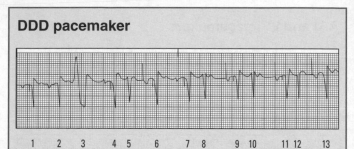

1 2 3   4 5   6   7 8   9 10   11 12   13

A dual-chamber pacemaker (with one lead in the atrium and another in the ventricle) provides versatile programming functions and can sense and pace in both the atrium and ventricle. This type of pacemaker mimics the normal cardiac cycle and maintains AV synchrony. It may be used for patients with chronic or intermittent AV block and for those who need atrial pacing or have delayed AV conduction or an increased risk of heart block.

When evaluating the rhythm strip of a patient with a DDD pacemaker, keep several points in mind:

• If the patient has an adequate intrinsic rhythm, the pacemaker won't fire; it doesn't need to.

• If you see an intrinsic P wave followed by a ventricular pacemaker spike, the pacemaker is tracking the atrial rate and assuring a ventricular response.

• If you see a pacemaker spike before a P wave, followed by an intrinsic ventricular QRS complex, the atrial rate is falling below the lower rate limit, causing the atrial channel to fire. Normal conduction to the ventricles follows.

• If you see a pacemaker spike before a P wave and before the QRS complex, no intrinsic activity is taking place in either the atria or ventricles.

The rhythm strip above shows the effects of a DDD pacemaker. Complexes 1, 2, 4, and 7 show the atrial-synchronous mode, set at a rate of 70. The patient has an intrinsic P wave, so the pacemaker only ensures that the ventricles respond. Complexes 3, 5, 8, 10, and 12 are intrinsic ventricular depolarizations. The pacemaker senses them and doesn't fire. In complexes 6, 9, and 11, the pacemaker is pacing the atria and ventricles in sequence. In complex 13, only the atria are paced; the ventricles respond on their own.

Asynchronous pacing modes
- Examples include AOO, VOO, and DOO.
- No sensing is involved; the pacemaker paces regardless of intrinsic impulses.
- The system provides pacing at a lower, programmed rate.
- Usually, this approach is used temporarily in pacemaker-dependent patients to ensure pacing during certain surgical and diagnostic procedures.

Through the ages

Pacemaker age considerations

Pacemakers in elderly patients
Older adults with active lifestyles who require pacemakers may respond best to AV synchronous pacemakers. That's because older adults have a greater reliance on atrial contraction, or atrial kick, to complete ventricular filling.

Pacemakers in pediatric patients
In a child, the demand rate of a programmable pacemaker can be set to a heart rate appropriate for the child's age. As the child grows, the heart rate can be adjusted to a lower rate.

Types of pacemakers

- A pacemaker can be permanent or temporary.
- Certain pacemakers pace both the left and right ventricles.

Permanent pacemaker

- A pacemaker may be implanted permanently when a patient has an arrhythmia, such as:
  - symptomatic bradyarrhythmia
  - tachyarrhythmia
  - sick sinus syndrome
  - varying degrees of AV block.

Biventricular pacemaker

- Used to treat patients with New York Heart Association class III or IV heart failure who have left ventricular dyssynchrony and would benefit from cardiac resynchronization therapy
- Uses traditional pacing leads in the right atrium and ventricle
- Adds a pacing lead for the left ventricle and additional pacemaker circuitry
- Has a specially designed lead for the left ventricle that's introduced through the coronary sinus and placed in a cardiac vein on surface of left ventricle (can be placed epicardially)
- Is a challenging implant for several reasons, including:
  - variable venous anatomy
  - contrast medium required to visualize cardiac veins
  - implant time longer than for typical pacemaker

I got myself a biventricular pacemaker because I wanted a chance to be a member of 'N Sync.

Placing a permanent pacemaker

Implanting a pacemaker is a simple surgical procedure performed with local anesthesia and moderate sedation. To implant an endocardial pacemaker, the cardiologist usually selects a transvenous route and begins lead placement by inserting a catheter percutaneously or by venous cutdown. Then, using fluoroscopic guidance, the surgeon threads the catheter through the vein until the tip reaches the endocardium.

Lead placement
For lead placement in the atrium, the tip must lodge in the right atrium or coronary sinus, as shown below. For placement in the ventricle, it must lodge in the right ventricular apex in one of the interior muscular ridges, or trabeculae (as shown below).

Implanting the generator
When the lead is in proper position, the cardiologist secures the pulse generator in a subcutaneous pocket of tissue just below the patient's clavicle. Changing the generator's battery or microchip circuitry requires only a shallow incision over the site and a quick exchange of components.

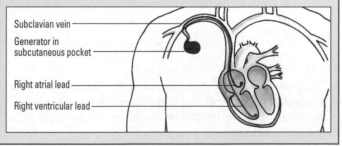

Subclavian vein

Generator in subcutaneous pocket

Right atrial lead

Right ventricular lead

- Delivers therapy every heartbeat (100% ventricular pacing), which:
  – coordinates ventricular contractions
  – improves hemodynamic status
  – paces QRS complexes (may be narrower or have different morphology than those associated with right ventricle pacing)

Biventricular lead placement

A biventricular pacemaker uses three leads: one to pace the right atrium, one to pace the right ventricle, and one to pace the left ventricle. The left ventricular lead is placed in the coronary sinus. Both ventricles are paced at the same time, causing them to contract simultaneously, which improves cardiac output.

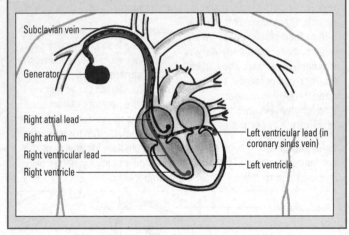

Temporary pacemaker

- Temporary pacemakers are commonly used in emergencies to support the patient until a permanent pacemaker is inserted or replaced or the problematic condition resolves. Indications include:
  - life-threatening bradyarrhythmias
  - evidence of decreased cardiac output (hypotension or syncope) after cardiac surgery
  - symptom-producing heart block
  - atrial or ventricular tachyarrhythmias that need overdrive pacing after cardiac surgery.
- These pacemakers may be invasive or noninvasive, but they don't require implantation.

- They have external pulse generators that are programmed by a touch pad or dials to control rate, output (in milliamperes, or mA), sensitivity, and AV interval.
- Several types of pacing can be performed: transvenous, epicardial, transcutaneous, and transthoracic.

Transvenous pacing

- Usually easily tolerated by the patient
- Most common and reliable type of temporary pacing

Characteristics of leadwires

- Balloon-tipped or stiff
- Inserted through subclavian, internal jugular, or femoral vein
- Advanced through a catheter into the right atrium or ventricle
- Connected to the pulse generator
- Inserted at the bedside or in a fluoroscopy suite

Characteristics of pulse generator

- Positive and negative poles, two sets for atrium and ventricle in dual-chamber models and one set for single-chamber pacing

Interventions after the pacing catheter is in place

- Measure threshold, and assess for capture.
- Set the rate, output, sensitivity, and mode.
- Perform paced ECG for documentation of pacing rhythm.
- Obtain chest X-ray to rule out pneumothorax and determine lead position.
- Maintain bed rest with limited progression of activity.

Epicardial pacing

- Used for patients undergoing cardiac surgery

Characteristics of leadwires

- Tips attached to heart surface
- Brought through chest wall below the incision
- Attached to the pulse generator
- Removed several days after surgery or when the patient no longer needs them

Temporary pulse generator

The settings on a temporary pulse generator may be changed in various ways to meet the patient's specific needs. The illustration below shows a single-chamber temporary pulse generator and gives brief descriptions of its various parts.

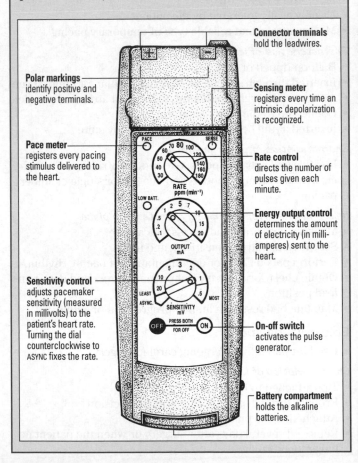

Connector terminals hold the leadwires.

Polar markings identify positive and negative terminals.

Sensing meter registers every time an intrinsic depolarization is recognized.

Pace meter registers every pacing stimulus delivered to the heart.

Rate control directs the number of pulses given each minute.

Energy output control determines the amount of electricity (in milliamperes) sent to the heart.

Sensitivity control adjusts pacemaker sensitivity (measured in millivolts) to the patient's heart rate. Turning the dial counterclockwise to ASYNC fixes the rate.

On-off switch activates the pulse generator.

Battery compartment holds the alkaline batteries.

Transcutaneous pacing

- Also known as *external pacing*
- Provides noninvasive VVI pacing
- Sends pacing impulses through the skin to the heart muscle
- Allows adjustment of rate and output (mA)
- Commonly used in emergencies until transvenous pacemakers can be inserted
- Variable patient tolerance
  - Keep sedatives and analgesia readily available.
  - Watch for skin irritation.

Positions of electrode pads

- Anterior-posterior placement (most common placement)
  - Place the anterior (front) electrode pad on the patient's anterior chest wall to the left of the sternum at the fourth and fifth intercostal spaces, halfway between the xiphoid process and left nipple.
  - Place the posterior (back) electrode pad on the left side of the back directly behind the anterior pad, just below the scapula to the left of the spine.
- Anterior-apex placement (alternative placement, if patient can't tolerate posterior placement)
  - Place the anterior (front) electrode pad on the patient's anterior chest wall to the left of the sternum at the fourth and fifth intercostal spaces, midaxillary line.
  - Place the posterior (back) electrode on the patient's anterior chest wall to the right of the upper sternum below the clavicle at the second or third intercostal space.

Transthoracic pacing

- Provides temporary ventricular pacing
- Used as a last resort during cardiac emergencies
- Requires insertion of a long needle into the right ventricle using subxiphoid approach
- Pacing wire is guided into the endocardium through the needle, and positive and negative terminals are attached to the pacemaker generator

Managing pacemaker therapy

Permanent pacemakers

- Use a systematic approach to assess pacemaker function for problems. Ask these questions:
  - What's the mode?
  - What are the lower and upper rate limits (maximum tracking or sensor rate)?
  - Are such features as mode switching or rate response activated?
  - Is the device a biventricular pacemaker?
  - Is the patient pacemaker-dependent?
  - Does the patient have signs and symptoms?
- Evaluate all sources of information, including:
  - patient identification card issued by the pacemaker manufacturer
  - patient history
  - patient or family knowledge of device function
  - doctor's notes, printouts from programmer if available
  - ECG observation.
- Review the patient's 12-lead ECG to evaluate pacemaker function. If unavailable, examine lead V_1 or MCL_1 instead.
- Select a monitoring lead that clearly shows the pacemaker spikes and compare at least two leads to verify what you observe.
- Remember that visibility of the spikes depends on pacing polarity, the type of lead, and the monitor's filter.
- Measure the rate and interpret the paced rhythm.
- Compare the morphology of paced and intrinsic complexes (traditional right ventricular pacing should produce a morphology similar to left bundle-branch block pattern).
- Differentiate between ventricular ectopy and paced activity.
- Look for information that tells you which chamber is paced and information about the pacemaker's sensing function.
- Monitor the patient's vital signs.

Distinguishing intermittent ventricular pacing from PVCs

Know whether your patient has an artificial pacemaker to help avoid mistaking a ventricular paced beat for a premature ventricular contraction (PVC). If your facility uses a monitoring system that eliminates artifact, make sure the monitor is set up correctly for a patient with a pacemaker. Otherwise, the pacemaker spikes may be eliminated as well.

If your patient has intermittent ventricular pacing, the paced ventricular complex will have a pacemaker spike preceding it, as shown in the shaded area of the top ECG strip below. You may need to look in different leads for a bipolar pacemaker spike because it's small and may be difficult to see. What's more, the paced ventricular complex of a properly functioning pacemaker won't occur prematurely; it will occur only when the patient's own ventricular rate falls below the rate set for the pacemaker.

If your patient is having PVCs, they'll occur prematurely and won't have pacemaker spikes preceding them. Examples are shown in the shaded areas of the bottom ECG strip.

Intermittent ventricular pacing

PVCs

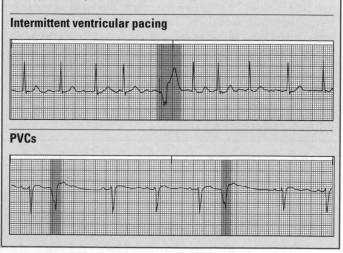

Assessing pacemaker function

When you apply a magnet to a pacemaker, the device reverts to a predefined (asynchronous) response mode that allows you to assess various aspects of pacemaker function. Specifically, you can:
• determine which chambers are being paced
• assess capture
• provide emergency pacing if the device malfunctions
• ensure pacing despite electromagnetic interference
• assess battery life by checking the magnet rate (a predetermined rate that indicates the need for battery replacement).

Keep in mind, however, that you must know which implanted device the patient has before you consider using a magnet on it. The patient might have an ICD, which only rarely is an appropriate target for magnet application.

It used to be relatively easy to tell a pacemaker from an ICD because of the difference in generator size and implant location. Now, however, the generators are similar in size, and both kinds of devices are implanted under the skin of the patient's chest. What's more, a single device may perform multiple functions.

In general, you shouldn't apply a magnet to an ICD or a pacemaker-ICD combination. Applying a magnet to an ICD can cause an unexpected response because various responses can be programmed in or determined by the manufacturer. When directed, applying a magnet to an ICD usually suspends therapies for ventricular tachycardia and fibrillation while leaving bradycardia pacing active, which may be helpful in patients who receive multiple, inappropriate shocks. Some models may beep when exposed to a magnetic field.

• Look for evidence of such problems as:
  – decreased cardiac output (hypotension, chest pain, dyspnea, syncope)
  – infection
  – pneumothorax

– misplaced electrode (abnormal electrical stimulation occurring in synchrony with the pacemaker, such as pectoral muscle twitching)
– stimulation of diaphragm (hiccups)
– cardiac tamponade.
• Placing a magnet over the pulse generator makes the pacemaker temporarily revert to an asynchronous mode (safety mode) at a preset rate.

Patient teaching
• Provide information to the patient about:
– function of pacemaker
– related anatomy and physiology
– patient's indication for pacemaker
– postoperative care and routines.
• Provide discharge instructions, including such topics as:
– incision care
– signs of pocket complications (hematoma, redness, swelling, purulent discharge, fever, bleeding)
– avoidance of heavy lifting or vigorous activity for 2 to 4 weeks
– limited arm movement on side of pacemaker for 2 to 3 months
– medical follow-up
– transtelephonic monitoring follow-up if indicated
– identification card to be carried
– procedure for taking pulse.
• Explain symptoms to report to doctor, including:
– light-headedness
– syncope
– fatigue
– palpitations
– muscle stimulation

Be sure to teach the patient everything he needs to know about his pacemaker.

- hiccups
- slow (below the base rate) or unusually fast heart rate.
- Because today's pacemakers are well shielded from environmental interactions, explain that the patient can safely use:
  - most common household appliances, including microwaves
  - cellular phones and bluetooth devices (on the side opposite the device)
  - spark-ignited combustion engines (such as on leaf blowers, lawnmowers, and automobiles)
  - office equipment (such as a computer, copier, fax machine)
  - light shop equipment.
- Caution the patient to avoid close or prolonged exposure to potential sources of electromagnetic interference (EMI).

Understanding EMI

EMI can wreak havoc on patients who have pacemakers or ICDs. For someone with a pacemaker, EMI may inhibit pacing, cause asynchronous or unnecessary pacing, or mimic intrinsic cardiac activity. For someone with an ICD, EMI may mimic ventricular fibrillation, or it may prevent detection of a problem that needs treatment.

If your patient has a pacemaker or an ICD, review common sources of EMI and urge the patient to avoid them. These may include:
- strong electromagnetic fields
- large generators and transformers
- arc and resistance welders
- large magnets
- motorized radiofrequency equipment
- large running engines or motors.

EMI may present a risk in medical or hospital settings as well. Make sure your patient knows to notify all health care providers about the implanted device so the provider can evaluate the risk of therapies such as:
- magnetic resonance imaging (usually contraindicated)
- radiation therapy (excluding diagnostic X-rays, such as mammograms, which typically are safe)
- diathermy
- electrocautery
- transcutaneous electrical nerve stimulation.

- Remind the patient about travel-related issues:
  – Metal detectors may disturb device function in a manner similar to that of a magnet.
  – Handheld scanning tools can be passed over the device but shouldn't linger over it.
  – An identification card may be needed to show security personnel.

Temporary pacemakers

- Check stimulation and sensing thresholds at least daily because they increase over time.
- Assess the patient and pacemaker regularly to check for possible problems, including:
  – failure to capture
  – undersensing
  – oversensing.
- Turn or reposition the patient carefully to prevent dislodgment of the leadwire.
- Follow recommended electrical safety precautions.
- Avoid microshocks to the patient by making sure that the bed and all electrical equipment are grounded properly and that all pacing wires and connections to temporary wires are secure and insulated with moisture-proof material (such as a disposable glove).
- If there's no output (pacing is required but the pacemaker fails to stimulate the heart), take the following steps:
  – Verify that the pacemaker is on.
  – Check the output and sensing settings.
  – Change the pulse generator battery.
  – Change the pulse generator.
  – Check for disconnection or dislodgment of the pacing wire.
- Obtain a chest X-ray and assist the doctor with repositioning the leadwire if required.
- All invasive temporary pacing has the potential to deliver a shock directly to the heart along the pacing wire, resulting in ventricular tachycardia or fibrillation.

- Defibrillation and cardioversion (up to 400 joules) don't usually require that the pulse generator be disconnected.
- Look for evidence of such problems as:
  – decreased cardiac output (hypotension, chest pain, dyspnea, syncope)
  – infection
  – pneumothorax
  – misplaced electrode (abnormal electrical stimulation occurring in synchrony with the pacemaker, such as pectoral muscle twitching)
  – stimulation of diaphragm (hiccups)
  – cardiac tamponade.

Patient teaching

- Provide information to the patient about:
  – function of pacemaker
  – related anatomy and physiology
  – patient's indication for pacemaker and potential need for permanent pacemaker
  – postprocedure care and pain management.
- Advise the patient not to get out of bed without assistance.
- Instruct the patient not to manipulate the pacemaker wires or pulse generator.
- Explain symptoms to report, including:
  – light-headedness
  – syncope
  – fatigue
  – palpitations
  – muscle stimulation
  – hiccups.
- Advise the patient to limit arm movement on the side of the pacemaker.

> The patient should limit arm movement on the side with the pacemaker.

Pacemaker problems

- A malfunctioning pacemaker can lead to arrhythmias, syncope, hypotension, and decreased cardiac output.
- Common causes of pacemaker problems include:
  - changes in the cardiac signal from MI or cardiomyopathy
  - disconnection or dislodgment of a lead
  - lead insulation failure
  - pulse generator failure (sensing circuits)
  - increased sensing threshold from edema or fibrosis at the electrode tip
  - reversion of pacemaker to asynchronous pacing.
- Pacemaker problems that can lead to low cardiac output and loss of AV synchrony include:
  - failure to capture
  - failure to pace
  - failure to sense (undersensing)
  - oversensing.

Failure to capture

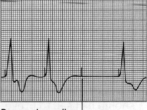

Pacemaker spike but no response from heart

- ECG shows a pacemaker spike without the appropriate atrial or ventricular response (spike without a complex).
- Patient may be asymptomatic or have signs of decreased cardiac output.
- Pacemaker can't stimulate the chamber.
- Problem may be caused by increased pacing thresholds related to certain situations, such as:
  - metabolic or electrolyte imbalance
  - antiarrhythmics
  - fibrosis or edema at electrode tip.
- Problem may be caused by lead malfunction, such as:
  - dislodged, fractured, or damaged lead

– perforation of myocardium by lead
– loose connection between lead and pulse generator.
- Related interventions may solve the problem, such as:
  – treating metabolic disturbance
  – replacing damaged leads
  – changing pulse generator battery
  – slowly increasing the output setting until capture occurs.

Failure to pace

- ECG shows no pacemaker activity when pacemaker activity should be evident.
- Magnet application yields no response (should cause asynchronous pacing).
- Problem has several common causes, including:
  – depleted battery
  – circuit failure
  – lead malfunction
  – inappropriate programming of sensing function
  – EMI.

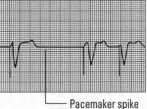

Pacemaker spike should appear here

- Failure to pace can lead to asystole or a severe decrease in cardiac output in pacemaker-dependent patients.
- If a pacemaker is failing to pace, a temporary pacemaker should be used to prevent asystole.
- Related interventions may solve the problem, such as:
  – replacing the pulse generator battery or pulse generator unit
  – adjusting the sensitivity setting
  – removing the source of EMI.

Failure to sense (undersensing)

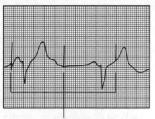

The pacemaker fires anywhere in the cycle

- ECG may show pacing spikes anywhere in cycle, including where intrinsic cardiac activity occurs.
- Patient may report feeling palpitations or skipped beats.
- Spikes on the T wave are especially dangerous because ventricular tachycardia or fibrillation may result.
- Problem has several common causes, including:
  - battery failure
  - fracture of pacing leadwire
  - displacement of electrode tip
  - "cross-talk" between atrial and ventricular channels
  - EMI mistaken for intrinsic signals.
- Related interventions may solve the problem, such as:
  - replacing the pulse generator battery or leadwires
  - adjusting the sensitivity setting.

Oversensing

- If the pacemaker is too sensitive, it can misinterpret muscle movement or extracardiac events as intrinsic cardiac electrical activity. As a result, pacing won't occur when it's needed.
- Pacing doesn't occur when the intrinsic rate drops below the lower set rate or pacing may not be observed in one or both chambers.
- AV synchrony can be lost.
- Problem has several common causes, including:
  - T-wave sensing
  - EMI
  - lead malfunction.
- Related interventions may solve the problem, such as:
  - adjusting the sensitivity setting
  - avoiding EMI
  - replacing the leadwire.

ICD basics

- Implanted electronic device that continually monitors the heart for bradycardia, VT, and VF and delivers shocks or paced beats to treat dangerous arrhythmias
- Used for life-threatening arrhythmias
- Programmed to detect many different arrhythmias
  - Ventricular tachycardia
  - Ventricular fibrillation
  - Bradycardia
  - Atrial fibrillation
- Automatically responds with appropriate therapy
- Widening indications over the past decade
- Implanted as primary prevention for patients at high risk for ventricular arrhythmias
  - Coronary disease and low ejection fraction
  - MI and impaired left ventricular systolic function
  - Dilated cardiomyopathy with low ejection fraction
  - Hypertrophic cardiomyopathy
  - Long QT syndrome and torsades de pointes
- Implanted as secondary prevention for patients who survive life-threatening arrhythmias
  - VF or hemodynamically unstable VT
  - Sustained VT with structural heart disease
- Detection rate
  - Defines what the device recognizes as ventricular tachycardia or fibrillation
  - Primary detection criterion
  - Has separate detection rates (zones) for ventricular tachycardia and ventricular fibrillation
  - Requires a rate sustained for a predetermined number of cycles
- Can deliver multitiered therapies
  - Defibrillation (always programmed)
  - Cardioversion (may be used for ventricular tachycardia)

– Antitachycardia pacing (may be used for ventricular tachycardia)
– Postshock pacing support (always programmed)
– Cardiac resynchronization therapy (also known as *biventricular pacing*)
– Bradycardia pacing

ICD review

An ICD has a programmable pulse generator and lead system that monitors the heart's activity, detects ventricular arrhythmias and other tachyarrhythmias, and responds with appropriate therapies. The range of therapies includes antitachycardia and antibradycardia pacing, cardioversion, and defibrillation. The ICD can also pace both the right atrium and right ventricle. Some can perform biventricular pacing. ICDs that provide therapy for atrial arrhythmias, such as atrial fibrillation, are also available.

Implantation of an ICD is similar to that of a permanent pacemaker. The cardiologist positions the lead (or leads) transvenously in the endocardium of the right ventricle (and the right atrium, if both chambers need pacing). The lead connects to a generator box implanted in the right or left upper chest near the clavicle.

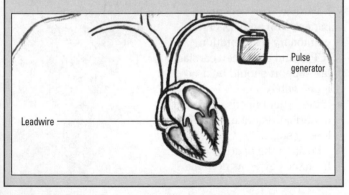

Pulse generator

Leadwire

Managing an ICD

- Know the device and how it's programmed, including:
  - type and model of ICD
  - status of the device (on or off)
  - detection rates
  - types of therapies that will be delivered and when.
- Evaluate the appropriateness of ICD shocks, including:
  - number of isolated and multiple shocks
  - situation and activity related to shocks
  - patient symptoms
  - ECG rhythm
  - drugs taken.
- Keep in mind that shocks may not occur despite ventricular tachycardia or fibrillation under certain circumstances, such as:
  - if the heart rate is less than the detection rate
  - if there's a lead or circuitry problem
  - if therapy is suspended or turned off
  - if the battery is depleted.
- If cardiac arrest occurs in a patient with an ICD, cardiopulmonary resuscitation (CPR) and advanced cardiac life support should be used immediately.
- If the patient needs external defibrillation, take the following steps:
  - Position the paddles as far from the device as possible.

> Mayday! ICD shocks may not occur when appropriate. Multiple shocks may also occur.

– Alternatively, use anterior-posterior position.

– Anticipate that defibrillation will result in "power on reset" and reversion to nominal settings.

– Programming of device should be verified with the programmer.

- Keep in mind that shocks can occur without ventricular tachycardia or fibrillation under certain circumstances, such as:

  – when the rate in sinus tachycardia ventures into the ventricular tachycardia zone

  – when noise is detected on the sensing lead (from electromagnetic interference or lead dysfunction)

  – when the patient develops atrial fibrillation.

- Keep in mind that multiple shocks may occur in certain circumstances, such as:

  – when the patient has persistent or recurrent ventricular tachycardia or fibrillation

  – when the device malfunctions.

- Multiple shocks indicate a medical emergency, and the patient may require adjunct treatment, such as:

  – CPR

  – external defibrillation

  – drugs such as amiodarone, lidocaine, procainamide

  – suspension of tachyarrhythmia therapy by magnet application or reprogramming of device.

- Look for evidence of problems, including:

  – decreased cardiac output (hypotension, chest pain, dyspnea, syncope)

  – infection

  – pneumothorax

  – misplaced electrode (abnormal electrical stimulation occurring in synchrony with the pacemaker, such as pectoral muscle twitching)

  – stimulation of diaphragm (hiccups)

  – cardiac tamponade.

Patient teaching

- Provide teaching similar to that for patients with pacemakers, plus additional teaching for special needs, such as:
  – patients who experienced cardiac arrest
  – patients still at risk for syncope
  – patients whose diagnoses may be associated with multiple life-changing components.
- Risk of syncope may continue because the device treats the arrhythmia but doesn't prevent ventricular tachycardia or fibrillation.
- Explain driving restrictions if ordered.
- Tell the patient and his family what to do if the device delivers a shock.
- Tell the patient what to do if symptoms of arrhythmia develop but the device doesn't deliver treatment:
  – Notify the doctor.
  – Activate local emergency medical service as appropriate.
  – Suggest training in CPR for family members.

Basic 12-lead electrocardiography

10

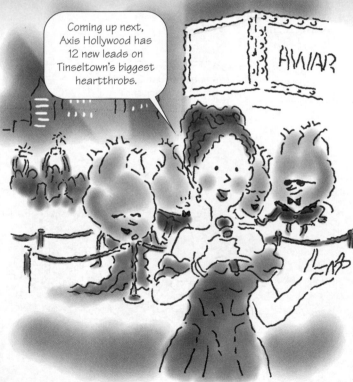

12-lead ECG fundamentals

- 12-lead ECG is a diagnostic test that serves several functions, including:
  – helping identify such pathologic conditions as myocardial ischemia and acute myocardial infarction (MI)
  – giving a more complete view of the heart's electrical activity than a rhythm strip
- Test results are viewed with other patient data, such as:
  – history
  – physical assessment findings
  – laboratory test results
  – diagnostic study results
  – drug regimen.

How does a 12-lead ECG get a better view of the heart? It goes out on a limb.

12-lead ECG leads

- In a 12-lead ECG, 12 leads provide 12 different views of the heart's electrical activity.
- Each lead transmits information about a different area of the heart.
- Waveforms obtained from each lead vary based on the location of the lead in relation to the depolarization wave passing through the myocardium.
- The 12 leads include six limb leads and six precordial leads.

Limb leads

- Record electrical activity in the heart's frontal plane (view through the middle of the heart from top to bottom and right to left)
- Include three bipolar limb leads (I, II, III)
- Include three unipolar augmented limb leads (aV_R, aV_L, and aV_F)

Precordial leads

- Also known as *chest leads*
- Provide information on electrical activity in the heart's horizontal plane (transverse view through the middle of the heart, dividing it into upper and lower portions)
- Include six unipolar leads (V_1, V_2, V_3, V_4, V_5, and V_6)
- Allow evaluation of left ventricle

Electrical axes

- Refer to the force and direction of the depolarization wave through the heart
- Recorded by a 12-lead ECG
- May be called the *mean QRS vector* or *mean instantaneous vector,* which refers to the mean of small electrical forces (instantaneous vectors) generated by impulses traveling through the heart
- In healthy hearts, are downward and to the left as a result of the impulse following a normal conduction pathway
- In unhealthy hearts, are variable and move away from areas of damage or necrosis and toward areas of hypertrophy

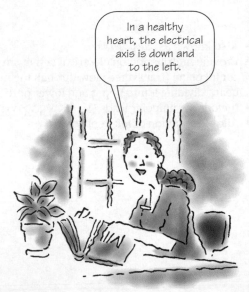

Electrical activity and the 12-lead ECG

Each of the leads on a 12-lead ECG views the heart from a different angle. These illustrations show the direction of electrical activity (depolarization) monitored by each lead and the 12 views of the heart.

Views reflected on a 12-lead ECG	Lead	View of the heart
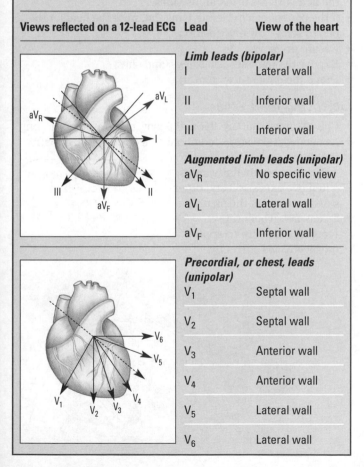	*Limb leads (bipolar)*	
	I	Lateral wall
	II	Inferior wall
	III	Inferior wall
	Augmented limb leads (unipolar)	
	aV_R	No specific view
	aV_L	Lateral wall
	aV_F	Inferior wall
	Precordial, or chest, leads (unipolar)	
	V_1	Septal wall
	V_2	Septal wall
	V_3	Anterior wall
	V_4	Anterior wall
	V_5	Lateral wall
	V_6	Lateral wall

Preparing for a 12-lead ECG

- Gather all needed supplies.
- Explain the procedure to the patient.
- Answer the patient's questions.
- Ask the patient to lie in a supine position in the center of the bed with his arms at his sides.
- If the patient can't tolerate lying flat, raise the head of the bed to semi-Fowler's position.
- Ensure privacy.
- Expose the patient's arms, legs, and chest.
- Drape the patient for comfort.

Selecting lead sites

- Choose areas that are flat and fleshy, not muscular or bony.
- As needed, take steps to enhance electrode contact with the skin:
  – Clip excessively hairy areas.
  – Remove excess oil and other substances from the skin.
- To ensure an accurate recording, be sure to apply the electrodes correctly.

> Picking a lead site is like pitching a tent. Look for a flat, soft terrain that's free from obstruction.

- Keep in mind that inaccurate placement of an electrode may lead to inaccurate waveforms and incorrect ECG interpretation.

Placing the leads

Limb leads

- Place electrodes on both of the patient's arms and on the left leg.
- Place an electrode on the right leg. (This is a ground that doesn't contribute to the waveform.)

Precordial leads

- Place the six unipolar precordial leads (V_1 through V_6) in sequence across the chest.

Through the ages

Obtaining a pediatric 12-lead ECG

You'll need patience when obtaining a 12-lead ECG from a pediatric patient. With the help of the parents, if possible, try distracting the attention of a young child. If artifact from arm and leg movement is a problem, place the electrodes in a more proximal position on the limb.

(Text continues on page 205.)

Limb lead placement

Proper lead placement is critical for accurate recording of cardiac rhythms. These drawings show correct electrode placement for the six limb leads. RA stands for right arm; LA, left arm; RL, right leg; and LL, left leg. A plus sign (+) indicates a positive pole, a minus sign (−) indicates a negative pole, and G indicates a ground. Below each drawing is a sample ECG strip for that lead.

Lead I
Connects the right arm (negative pole) with the left arm (positive pole).

Lead II
Connects the right arm (negative pole) with the left leg (positive pole).

Lead III
Connects the left arm (negative pole) with the left leg (positive pole).

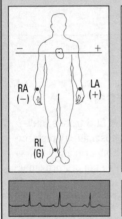

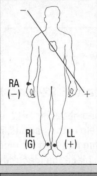

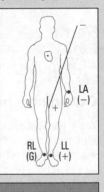

Limb lead placement *(continued)*

Lead aV_R

Lead aV_R
Connects the right arm (positive pole) with the heart (negative pole).

Lead aV_L
Connects the left arm (positive pole) with the heart (negative pole)

Lead aV_F
Connects the left leg (positive pole) with the heart (negative pole).

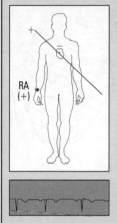

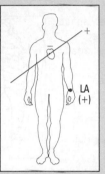

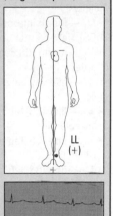

Precordial lead placement

To record a 12-lead ECG, place electrodes on the patient's arms and left leg and place a ground lead on the patient's right leg. The three standard limb leads (I, II, and III) and the three augmented leads (aV_R, aV_L, and aV_F) are recorded using these electrodes. Then, to record the precordial chest leads, place electrodes as follows:

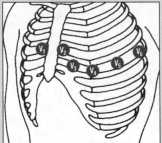

- V_1—fourth intercostal space (ICS), right sternal border
- V_2—fourth ICS, left sternal border
- V_3—midway between V_2 and V_4
- V_4—fifth ICS, left mid-clavicular line
- V_5—fifth ICS, left anterior axillary line
- V_6—fifth ICS, left midaxillary line.

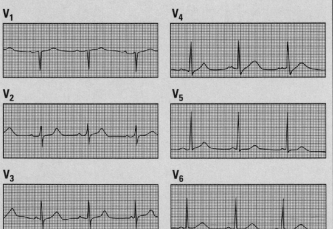

V_1 V_4

V_2 V_5

V_3 V_6

Leads used with 12-lead ECG

- Two additional lead types may be used with 12-lead ECG for diagnostic purposes.
- These leads assess areas that a standard 12-lead ECG can't.

Right precordial leads

- Six unipolar leads (V_{1R}, V_{2R}, V_{3R}, V_{4R}, V_{5R}, and V_{6R})
- Allows evaluation of the right ventricle

Posterior leads

- Three unipolar leads (V_7, V_8, and V_9)
- Allows assessment of the posterior surface of the heart

Hey, I'm a shy guy. I'm not sure if I want anyone looking at my posterior.

(Text continues on page 208.)

Right precordial lead placement

Right precordial leads can provide specific information about the function of the right ventricle. Place the six leads on the right side of the chest in a mirror image of the standard precordial lead placement, as shown here:

V_{1R} — fourth intercostal space (ICS), left sternal border
V_{2R} — fourth ICS, right sternal border
V_{3R} — halfway between V_{2R} and V_{4R}
V_{4R} — fifth ICS, right midclavicular line
V_{5R} — fifth ICS, right anterior axillary line
V_{6R} — fifth ICS, right midaxillary line.

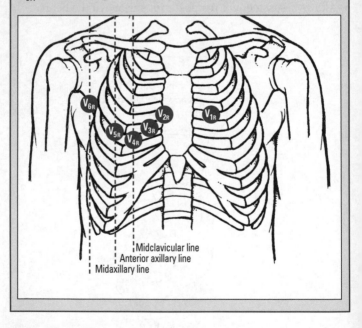

Midclavicular line
Anterior axillary line
Midaxillary line

Posterior lead placement

Posterior leads can be used to assess the posterior side of the heart. To ensure an accurate reading, make sure the posterior electrodes V_7, V_8, and V_9 are placed at the same horizontal level as the V_6 lead at the fifth intercostal space. Place lead V_7 at the posterior axillary line, lead V_9 at the paraspinal line, and lead V_8 halfway between leads V_7 and V_9.

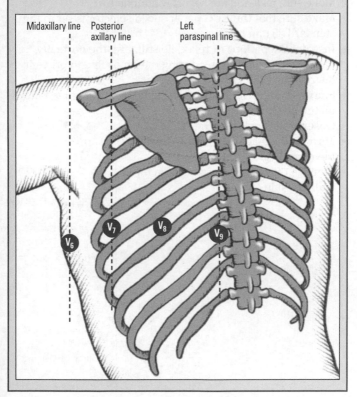

Recording the ECG

- Plug the cord of the ECG machine into a grounded outlet unless the machine operates on a charged battery and doesn't need to be plugged in.
- Turn on the machine.
- Enter the patient's identification data if necessary.
- Place all of the electrodes on the patient.
- Make sure all leads are securely attached.
- Make sure that the ECG paper speed selector is set to the standard 25 mm per second.
- Instruct the patient to relax, lie still, breathe normally, and refrain from talking during the recording to prevent distortion of the ECG tracing.
- Start recording the ECG by pressing the appropriate button on the machine.
- Observe the quality of the tracing.
- Turn off the machine when it finishes the recording.
- Remove the electrodes and clean the patient's skin.

Memory jogger

GO SLOW to remember the steps for recording an ECG:

Grounded outlet

On (machine and electrodes)

Speed (25 mm/sec)

Lie still (instruction to the patient)

Observe tracing quality

Wash the patient's skin after removing the electrodes.

Reading the ECG

- Make sure the printout shows pertinent information, including:
  - patient's name
  - patient's room number
  - patient's medical record number if appropriate
  - date
  - time
  - doctor's name
  - patient's heart rate
  - wave durations (measured in seconds)
  - lead that's being recorded.
- Make sure special circumstances (such as those listed here) are noted:
  - episodes of chest pain
  - abnormal electrolyte levels
  - related drug treatment
  - abnormal placement of electrodes
  - presence of an artificial pacemaker
  - whether a magnet was used while the ECG was obtained.
- Keep in mind these important facts about ECG recordings:
  - They're legal documents.
  - They belong in the patient's medical record.
  - They must be saved for future reference and comparison with baseline strips.

Understanding a multichannel ECG recording

The top of a 12-lead ECG recording typically includes patient identification information and an interpretation by the machine. A rhythm strip commonly appears at the bottom of the recording.

On the recording, look for standardization marks, normally 10 small squares in height. If the patient has high-voltage complexes, the marks will be one-half as high. You'll also notice that lead markers separate the lead recordings on the paper and that each lead is named.

Familiarize yourself with the way the leads are laid out on the recording so you can interpret the ECG results more quickly and accurately.

Patient and   Rhythm   Lead   Lead   Standardization
ECG information   strip   marker   name   mark

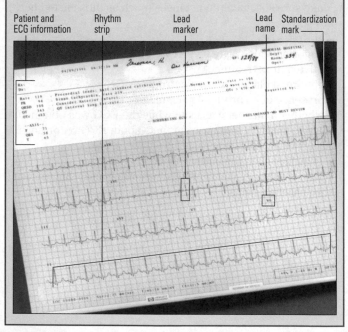

Advanced electrocardiography

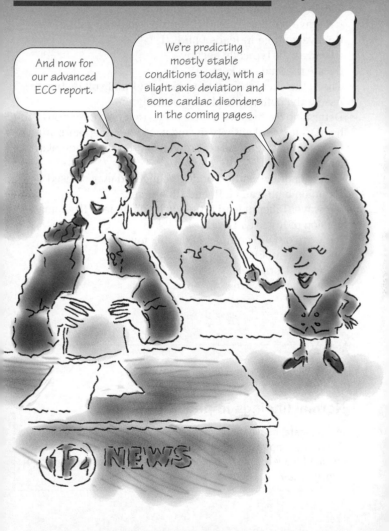

Steps in ECG interpretation

- Check the ECG tracing to see if it's technically correct.
- Use a systematic approach for interpretation, and compare the current ECG with the patient's previous ECG.
- Quickly scan limb leads I, II, and III:
  - R-wave voltage in lead II should equal the sum of the R-wave voltage in leads I and III.
  - Lead aV_R is typically negative.
- Locate the lead markers.
- Check the standardization markings (1 millivolt or 10 mm).
- Assess the patient's heart rate and rhythm.
- Determine the heart's electrical axis (average direction of the heart's electrical activity during ventricular depolarization):
  - Examine waveforms recorded from the six frontal plane leads: I, II, III, aV_R, aV_L, and aV_F.
  - The quadrant method or degree method may be used.
- Examine limb leads I, II, and III:
  - R wave: Taller in lead II than in lead I; in lead III, a smaller version of R wave in lead I
  - P wave or QRS complex: Possibly inverted
  - ST segment: Flat
  - T wave: Upright
  - Pathologic Q waves: Absent

Through the ages

Normal findings in pediatric ECGs

In a neonate, dominant R waves in the chest leads and upright T waves are normal findings. By the end of the first week of life, the T wave in lead V_1 becomes inverted and remains inverted through age 7.

R-wave progression

R waves should progress normally through the precordial leads. Note that the R wave in this strip is the first positive deflection in the QRS complex. Also note that the S wave gets smaller, or regresses, from lead V_1 to V_6 until it finally disappears.

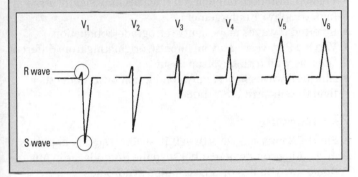

- Examine limb leads aV_R, aV_L, and aV_F:
  – Leads aV_L and aV_F: Possibly similar tracings but lead aV_F should have taller P and R waves
  – P wave, QRS complex, and T wave: Deflect downward in lead aV_R
- Examine the R wave in the precordial leads:
  – Progressively taller from lead V_1 to V_5
  – Slightly smaller in lead V_6
- Examine the S wave in the precordial leads:
  – Extremely deep in lead V_1
  – Progressively more shallow
  – Usually gone by lead V_5

Waveform abnormalities

- The location of changes in each lead can determine the area of the heart affected.

P waves

- Peaked, notched, or enlarged P waves may signify atrial hypertrophy or enlargement.
- Inverted P waves may signify retrograde conduction.
- Varying P waves signify an impulse originating from different sites, as with irritable atrial tissue.
- Absent P waves may signify conduction by a route other than the sinoatrial (SA) node.

PR intervals

- Short PR intervals (less than 0.12 second) signify impulses originating somewhere other than the SA node, as in junctional arrhythmias or preexcitation syndromes.
- Prolonged PR intervals (greater than 0.20 second) signify a conduction delay, as in heart block or digoxin toxicity.

QRS complex

- A duration greater than 0.12 second may signify ventricular conduction.
- One or more missing QRS complexes may signify atrioventricular (AV) block or ventricular standstill.

Q wave

- A Q wave is considered abnormal if it has a depth greater than 4 mm or a height of one-fourth of the R wave.
- Abnormal Q waves signify myocardial necrosis.
- Abnormal Q waves develop when damaged tissue prevents depolarization from following its normal path.

ST segment

- The ST segment is considered abnormal if it's elevated more than 1 mm above the baseline, depressed more than 0.5 mm below the baseline, or both.
- It will be elevated in leads facing an injured area.
- It will be depressed in leads facing away from the injured area.

T wave

- Tall, peaked, or tented T waves may signify myocardial injury or hyperkalemia.
- Inverted T waves may signify myocardial ischemia.

QT interval

- A prolonged QT interval (greater than 0.44 second) indicates prolonged ventricular repolarization and congenital prolonged QT syndrome.
- A short QT interval (less than 0.36 second) may result from digoxin toxicity or hypercalcemia.

> Waveform abnormalities are clues to the location of the affected area of the heart.

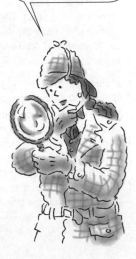

Electrical axis deviation

- Finding the patient's electrical axis can help confirm a diagnosis.
- Axis deviation occurs when electrical activity in the heart moves away from areas of damage or necrosis.
- Normal: Between 0 and 90 degrees (some sources consider −30 to 90 degrees normal)
- Right axis deviation: Between 90 and 180 degrees
- Left axis deviation: Between 0 and −90 degrees (some sources consider −30 to −90 degrees left axis deviation)
- Extreme right axis deviation (indeterminate axis): Between −180 and −90 degrees

Hexaxial reference system

The hexaxial reference system consists of six bisecting lines (each represents one of the six limb leads) and a circle that represents the heart. The intersection of all lines divides the circle into equal, 30-degree segments.

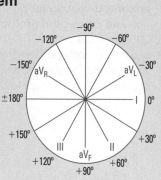

Shifting degrees

Note that 0 degrees appears at the 3 o'clock position (positive pole lead I). Moving counterclockwise, the degrees become increasingly negative until reaching ±180 degrees at the 9 o'clock position (negative pole lead I).

The bottom half of the circle contains the corresponding positive degrees. However, a positive-degree designation doesn't necessarily mean that the pole is positive.

(Text continues on page 219.)

Electrical axis determination: Quadrant method

This chart will help you quickly determine the direction of a patient's electrical axis. Observe the deflections of the QRS complexes in leads I and aV_F. Lead I indicates whether impulses are moving to the right or left, and lead aV_F indicates whether they're moving up or down. Then check the chart to determine whether the patient's axis is normal or has a left, right, or extreme right axis deviation.

- Normal axis: QRS-complex deflection is positive or upright in both leads.
- Left axis deviation: Lead I is upright and lead aV_F points down.
- Right axis deviation: Lead I points down and lead aV_F is upright.
- Extreme right axis deviation: Both waves point down.

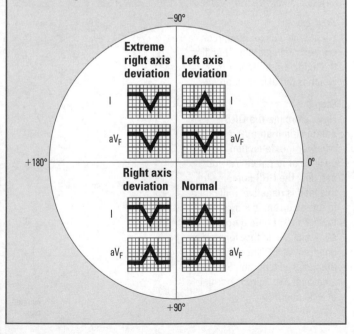

Electrical axis determination: Degree method

The degree method provides a more precise, exact measurement of the electrical axis. It allows you to identify a patient's electrical axis by degrees on the hexaxial system, not just by quadrant. It also allows you to determine the axis even if the QRS complex isn't clearly positive or negative in leads I and aV$_F$. To use this method, take the following steps.

Step 1
Identify the limb lead with the smallest QRS complex or the equiphasic QRS complex. In this example, it's lead III.

Lead I	Lead II	Lead III	Lead aV$_R$	Lead aV$_L$	Lead aV$_F$

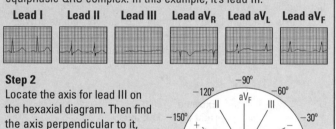

Step 2
Locate the axis for lead III on the hexaxial diagram. Then find the axis perpendicular to it, which is the axis for lead aV$_R$.

Step 3
Now, examine the QRS complex in lead aV$_R$, noting whether the deflection is positive or negative. As you can see, the QRS complex for this lead is negative, indicating that the current is moving toward the negative pole of aV$_R$, which is in the right lower quadrant at +30 degrees on the hexaxial diagram. So the electrical axis here is normal at +30 degrees.

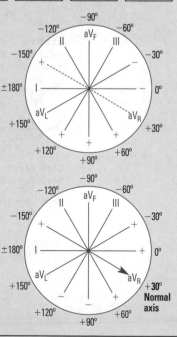

Causes of axis deviation

- Factors that influence axis location include the position of the heart in the chest, heart size, body size, and conduction pathways.
- Deviation isn't always cardiac in origin, and it isn't always an abnormality. For example, infants and children normally have right axis deviation and pregnant women normally have left axis deviation.

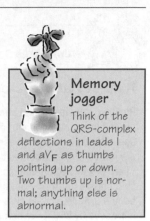

Memory jogger
Think of the QRS-complex deflections in leads I and aV$_F$ as thumbs pointing up or down. Two thumbs up is normal; anything else is abnormal.

Left axis deviation

- May be a normal variation
- Causes
  - Aging
  - Aortic stenosis
  - Inferior-wall myocardial infarction (MI)
  - Left anterior hemiblock
  - Left bundle-branch block (LBBB)
  - Left ventricular hypertrophy
  - Mechanical shifts (ascites, pregnancy, tumors)
  - Wolff-Parkinson-White (WPW) syndrome

Right axis deviation

- May be a normal variation
- Causes
  - Emphysema
  - Lateral-wall MI
  - Left posterior hemiblock
  - Pulmonary hypertension
  - Pulmonic stenosis
  - Right bundle-branch block (RBBB)
  - Right ventricular hypertrophy

Through the ages

Axis deviation across the life span

Right axis deviation, between +60 degrees and +160 degrees, is normal in neonates due to dominance of the right ventricle. By age 1, the axis falls between +10 degrees and +100 degrees as the left ventricle becomes dominant.

Left axis deviation commonly occurs in elderly people. This axis shift may result from fibrosis of the anterior fascicle of the left bundle branch or thickness of the left ventricular wall, which increases by 25% between ages 30 and 80.

Read on to find out how disorders can affect ECGs.

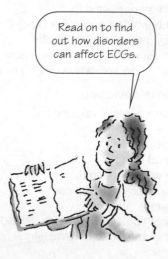

Disorder-related 12-lead ECG changes

Angina

- A symptom of myocardial ischemia
- Occurs when the myocardium needs more oxygen than the coronary arteries can deliver

Stable angina

- Provoked by exertion or stress
- Usually lasts 2 to 10 minutes
- Typically relieved by rest
- Repeats in this pattern

Unstable angina

- Provoked more easily than stable angina
- Commonly wakes the patient
- Unpredictable
- Worsens over time
- Classified as an acute coronary syndrome with MI
- Treated as a medical emergency
- Usually signals an MI

ECG changes in angina

Some classic ECG changes involving the T wave and ST segment that you may see when monitoring a patient with angina are illustrated below.

Peaked T wave	Flattened T wave	T-wave inversion	ST-segment depression with T-wave inversion	ST-segment depression without T-wave inversion

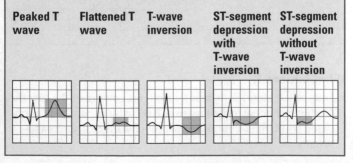

Prinzmetal's angina
- A relatively uncommon form of unstable angina
- Usually occurs at rest or wakes the patient from sleep

ECG changes in Prinzmetal's angina

This illustration shows a 12-lead ECG of a patient with Prinzmetal's angina. Marked ST-segment elevations appear in leads that are monitoring the heart area where the coronary artery spasm occurs. The elevation occurs during chest pain and resolves when pain subsides. T waves are usually of normal size and configuration.

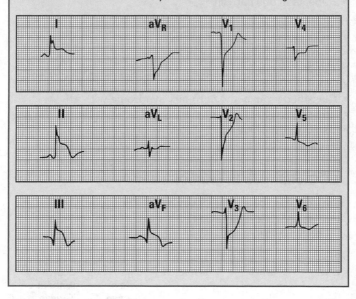

What causes it
- Decreased blood flow results from narrowing of the arteries from coronary artery disease (CAD), which may be complicated by platelet clumping, thrombus formation, or vasospasm.

- In Prinzmetal's angina, vasospasm results from a focal episodic spasm of a coronary artery, with or without an obstructing coronary artery lesion.

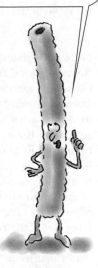

When I become too narrow-minded, it can be bad news for the whole cardiovascular system.

What to look for

Stable angina
- Predictable pain pattern
- Substernal or precordial burning, squeezing, or tightness
- May radiate to left arm, neck, or jaw
- Relieved by nitrates or rest

Unstable angina
- Chest pain that may radiate
- Greater intensity and duration than stable angina
- Also pallor, diaphoresis, nausea, or anxiety

Prinzmetal's angina
- Substernal chest pain from heaviness to crushing discomfort
- Usually occurs at rest or wakes the patient from sleep
- Also dyspnea, nausea, vomiting, or diaphoresis

How it's treated

- Give nitrates to reduce myocardial oxygen consumption.
- Give beta-adrenergic blockers to reduce the heart's workload and oxygen demands.
- Give calcium channel blockers to treat angina caused by coronary artery spasm.
- Give antiplatelet drugs to minimize platelet aggregation and the risk of coronary occlusion.
- Give antilipemic drugs to reduce elevated serum cholesterol or triglyceride levels.

- If the patient has continued unstable angina or acute chest pain or has had an invasive cardiac procedure, give glycoprotein IIb/IIIa inhibitors to reduce platelet aggregation.
- Anticipate coronary artery bypass surgery (CABG) or percutaneous transluminal coronary angioplasty (PTCA) for obstructive lesions.

Myocardial infarction

- MI is categorized as an acute coronary syndrome.
- Reduced blood flow through one or more coronary arteries causes myocardial ischemia and necrosis.
- Damage usually occurs in the left ventricle, although the location varies with the coronary artery affected.
- As long as the myocardium is deprived of oxygen-rich blood, the ECG will reflect three pathologic changes: ischemia, injury, and infarction.
- In a non-ST-segment-elevation MI, abnormalities may include no ST-segment elevation or ST-segment depression.
- In an ST-segment-elevation MI, abnormalities may include ST-segment elevation and significant Q waves, which represent scarring and necrosis.

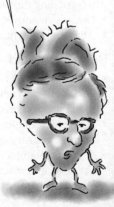

My oh my-o my! A lack of oxygen can damage the myocardium and cause MI.

(Text continues on page 227.)

Zones of MI

MI is characterized by a central area of necrosis surrounded by a zone of injury that may recover if revascularization occurs. This zone of injury is surrounded by an outer zone of reversible ischemia. Each zone produces characteristic ECG changes.

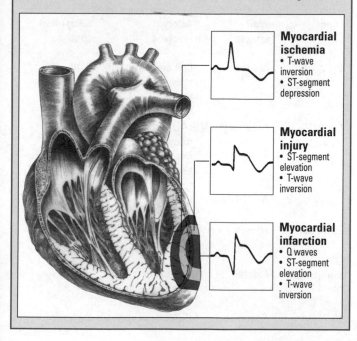

Myocardial ischemia
• T-wave inversion
• ST-segment depression

Myocardial injury
• ST-segment elevation
• T-wave inversion

Myocardial infarction
• Q waves
• ST-segment elevation
• T-wave inversion

Locating myocardial damage

After you've noted characteristic lead changes (ST elevation, abnormal Q waves) in an acute MI, use this table to identify the areas of damage, the affected wall, and the artery involved. The last column shows reciprocal lead changes.

Leads	Wall affected	Artery involved	Reciprocal changes
V_2, V_3, V_4	Anterior	Left coronary, left anterior descending (LAD)	II, III, aV_F
I, aV_L, V_2, V_3, V_4 V_5, V_6	Anterolateral	LAD and diagonal branches, circumflex and marginal branches	II, III, aV_F
V_1, V_2, V_3, V_4	Anteroseptal	LAD	None
II, III, aV_F	Inferior	Right coronary (RCA)	I, aV_L
I, aV_L, V_5, V_6	Lateral	Circumflex branch of left coronary	II, III, aV_F
V_8, V_9	Posterior	RCA or circumflex	V_1, V_2, V_3, V_4 (R greater than S in V_1 and V_2, ST-segment depression, elevated T wave)
V_{4R}, V_{5R}, V_{6R}	Right ventricular	RCA	None

What causes it

- Atherosclerosis
  - Formation of plaque, an unstable and lipid-rich substance
  - Subsequent rupture or erosion of plaque, resulting in platelet adhesion, fibrin clot formation, and activation of thrombin
- Embolus

Risk factors

- Diabetes
- Family history of heart disease
- High-fat, high-carbohydrate diet
- Hyperlipoproteinemia
- Hypertension
- Menopause
- Obesity
- Sedentary lifestyle
- Smoking
- Stress

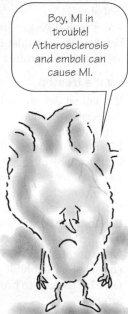

Boy, MI in trouble! Atherosclerosis and emboli can cause MI.

What to look for

- ECG changes
  - ST-segment elevation or depression
  - Abnormal Q waves
  - T wave inversion
- Chest pain
  - Severe, persistent, burning, squeezing, or crushing
  - Usually substernal or precordial
  - May radiate to left arm, neck, jaw, or shoulder blade
  - Lasts at least 20 minutes and may persist for several hours
  - Unrelieved by rest
- Anxiety
- Cool extremities
- Fatigue
- Feeling of impending doom

- Hypertension
- Hypotension
- Nausea and vomiting
- Shortness of breath
- Atypical presentation
  – More likely in women, elderly patients, and patients with diabetes
  – May include vague or absent chest discomfort, back pain between the shoulder blades, shortness of breath, fatigue, or abdominal discomfort

How it's treated

- If a patient develops chest pain, take immediate measures to decrease cardiac workload and increase oxygen supply to the myocardium.
- If symptoms started during the previous 12 hours, prepare for thrombolytic therapy (unless contraindicated) to restore vessel patency and minimize necrosis in ST-segment-elevation MI.
- Give oxygen to increase oxygenation of blood.
- Give nitroglycerin sublingually to relieve chest pain (unless systolic blood pressure is less than 90 mm Hg).
- Give morphine to relieve pain.
- Give aspirin to inhibit platelet aggregation.
- Give I.V. heparin to promote patency in the affected coronary artery.
- If the patient has an arrhythmia, prepare for use of anti-arrhythmics, transcutaneous pacing patches (or transvenous pacemaker), defibrillation, or epinephrine.
- A patient without hypotension, bradycardia, or excessive tachycardia may receive I.V. nitroglycerin for 24 to 48 hours to reduce afterload and preload and relieve chest pain.
- If the patient has continued unstable angina or acute chest pain or has had an invasive cardiac procedure, give glycoprotein IIb/IIIa inhibitors to reduce platelet aggregation.

- Give angiotensin-converting enzyme inhibitors to reduce preload and afterload and prevent remodeling (begin 6 hours after admission, or when stable, in ST-segment-elevation MI).
- PTCA, stent placement, or CABG may be used to open blocked or narrowed arteries.

(Text continues on page 234.)

Recognizing an anterior-wall MI

This 12-lead ECG shows typical characteristics (V_2, V_3, V_4) of an anterior-wall MI. Note that the R waves don't progress through the precordial leads. Also note the ST-segment elevation in leads V_2 and V_3. As expected, the reciprocal leads II, III, and aV_F show slight ST-segment depression.

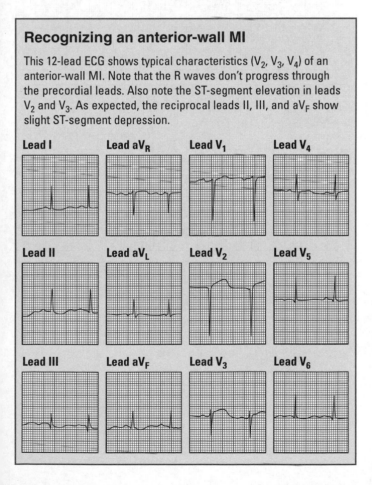

Recognizing an anteroseptal-wall MI

This 12-lead ECG shows typical characteristics of an anteroseptal-wall MI. Note the loss of R wave in leads V_1 and V_2. Also note the ST-segment elevation in leads V_1 to V_4.

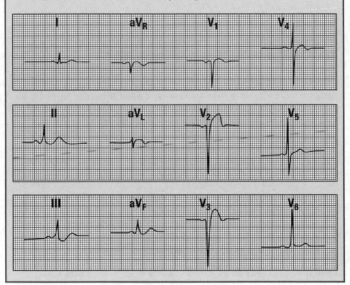

Recognizing an inferior-wall MI

This 12-lead ECG shows the characteristic changes of an inferior-wall MI. In leads II, III, and aV$_F$, note the T-wave inversion, ST-segment elevation, and pathologic Q waves. In leads I and aV$_L$, note the slight ST-segment depression — a reciprocal change.

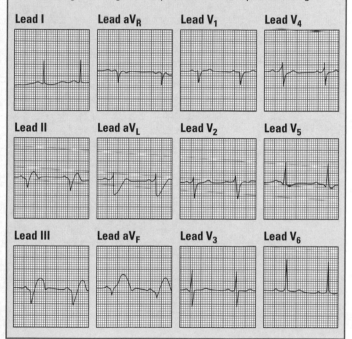

Recognizing a lateral-wall MI

This 12-lead ECG shows typical characteristics of a lateral-wall MI. Note the ST-segment elevation in leads I, aV$_L$, V$_5$, and V$_6$.

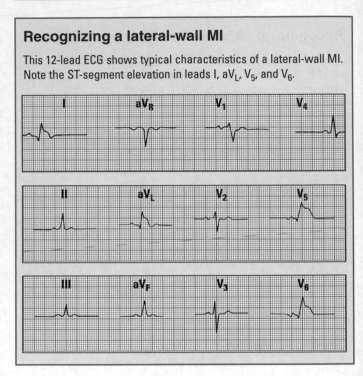

Recognizing a right-ventricular-wall MI

This 12-lead ECG shows typical traits of a right-ventricular-wall MI. Note the ST-segment elevation in the right precordial chest leads (V_{4R}, V_{5R}, and V_{6R}). Pathologic Q waves may also appear in leads V_{4R}, V_{5R}, and V_{6R}.

Left-side leads   **Right-side leads**

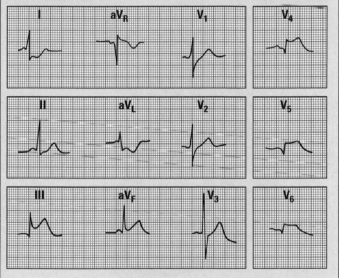

Reciprocal changes in MI

Ischemia, injury, and infarction—the three I's of MI—produce characteristic ECG changes. The changes shown by leads that reflect electrical activity facing the damaged areas are shown to the right of the illustration below. Reciprocal leads, those opposite the damaged area, show opposing ECG changes, as shown to the left of the illustration.

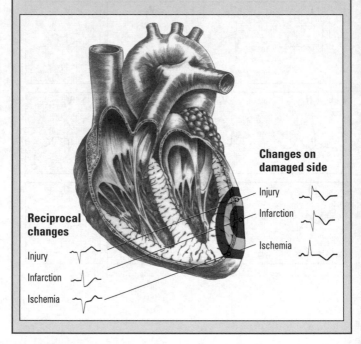

Changes on damaged side

Injury

Infarction

Ischemia

Reciprocal changes

Injury

Infarction

Ischemia

Pericarditis

- Inflammation of the pericardium (fibroserous sac that envelops the heart)

Acute pericarditis

- May be fibrinous or effusive
- May include purulent, serous, or hemorrhagic exudates

Chronic pericarditis
- Causes dense fibrous thickening of the pericardium

What causes it
- Autoimmune disorders
- Bacterial, fungal, or viral disorders
- Complications of cardiac injury (MI, cardiotomy)
- High-dose radiation therapy to the chest
- Rheumatic fever

What to look for
Acute pericarditis
- Arrhythmias
- Chest pain that typically worsens with deep inspiration and improves when the patient sits up and leans forward
- Chills
- Diaphoresis
- Dyspnea
- Fever
- Pericardial friction rub

Chronic pericarditis
- Symptoms similar to those of chronic right-sided heart failure (edema, ascites, and hepatomegaly)
- Palpable, sometimes audible, sharp knock or rub in early diastole, when the rapidly filling ventricle touches the unexpansive pericardium

> Signs and symptoms of acute pericarditis include arrhythmias, chest pain, chills, sweating, dyspnea, and fever.

Recognizing pericarditis

ECG changes in acute pericarditis evolve through two stages:
• Stage 1—Diffuse ST-segment elevations of 1 to 2 mm in most limb leads and most precordial leads reflect the inflammatory process. Upright T waves appear in most leads. The ST-segment and T-wave changes are typically seen in leads I, II, III, aV$_R$, aV$_F$, and V$_2$ through V$_6$.
• Stage 2—As pericarditis resolves, the ST-segment elevation and accompanying T-wave inversion resolves in most leads.

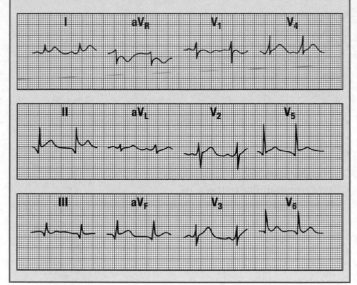

How it's treated
• Identification and treatment of the underlying cause

Acute pericarditis
• Maintain bed rest and administer corticosteroids or nonsteroidal anti-inflammatory drugs to relieve pain and inflammation.

Infectious pericarditis
- Administer antibiotics to fight infection.

Cardiac tamponade
- Assist with pericardiocentesis to remove fluid from around the heart.

Constrictive pericarditis
- Prepare the patient for complete pericardiectomy to allow fluid to drain from around the heart.

Comparing MI with acute pericarditis

MI and acute pericarditis each cause ST-segment elevation on an ECG. However, the ST segment and T wave (shaded areas below) on an MI waveform are quite different from those on a pericarditis waveform. Also, because pericarditis involves the surrounding pericardium, several leads show ST-segment and T-wave changes (typically leads I, II, III, aV$_L$, aV$_F$, and V$_2$ through V$_6$). In an MI, only leads reflecting the area of infarction show the characteristic changes.

Myocardial infarction

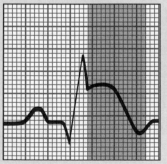

Acute pericarditis

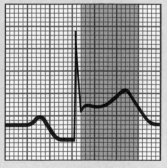

Left ventricular hypertrophy

- Characterized by a thickened left ventricular wall
- Results from conditions that cause chronically increased pressure in the ventricle
- May lead to left-sided heart failure and subsequent changes
  - Increased left atrial pressure
  - Pulmonary vascular congestion
  - Pulmonary arterial hypertension
- May decrease coronary artery perfusion, causing an MI
- May alter the papillary muscle, causing mitral insufficiency

What causes it

- Aortic stenosis or insufficiency
- Cardiomyopathy
- Mitral insufficiency
- Systemic hypertension (most common)

What to look for

- Signs and symptoms related to the underlying disorder

Recognizing left ventricular hypertrophy

Left ventricular hypertrophy can lead to heart failure or MI. The rhythm strips shown here illustrate key ECG changes of left ventricular hypertrophy as they occur in selected leads: a large S wave (shaded area in left strip) in V_1 and a large R wave

Lead V_1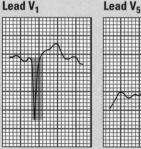

Lead V_5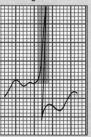

(shaded area in right strip) in V_5. If the depth (in mm) of the S wave in V_1 added to the height (in mm) of the R wave in V_5 exceeds 35 mm, then the patient has left ventricular hypertrophy.

How it's treated

- Interventions focus on proper management of the underlying disorder, such as hypertension.

Bundle-branch block

- A potential complication of MI
- Characterized by abnormal impulse conduction through the left or right bundle branch that results in a QRS complex longer than 0.12 second
- May be difficult to differentiate between BBB and WPW syndrome

What causes it

RBBB

- MI
- CAD
- Pulmonary embolism
- Increased heart rate (rate-related RBBB)

LBBB

- Hypertensive heart disease
- Aortic stenosis
- Degenerative changes of the conduction system
- CAD
- MI

What to look for

- ECG changes in the QRS complex (changes in configuration, duration greater than 0.12 second) and T-wave changes

How it's treated

- BBB may be treated with a temporary pacemaker.
- Monitor to detect progression to a more complete block.

Understanding RBBB

In RBBB, the initial impulse activates the interventricular septum from left to right, just as in normal activation (arrow 1). Next, the left bundle branch activates the left ventricle (arrow 2). The impulse then crosses the interventricular septum to activate the right ventricle (arrow 3).

In this disorder, the QRS complex exceeds 0.12 second and has a different configuration, sometimes resembling rabbit ears or the letter "M." Septal depolarization isn't affected in lead V_1, so the initial small R wave remains.

The R wave is followed by an S wave, which represents left ventricular depolarization, and a tall R wave (called R prime, or R'), which represents late right ventricular depolarization. The T wave is negative in this lead; however, the negative deflection is called a secondary T-wave change and isn't clinically significant.

The opposite occurs in lead V_6. A small Q wave is followed by depolarization of the left ventricle, which produces a tall R wave. Depolarization of the right ventricle then causes a broad S wave. In lead V_6, the T wave should be positive.

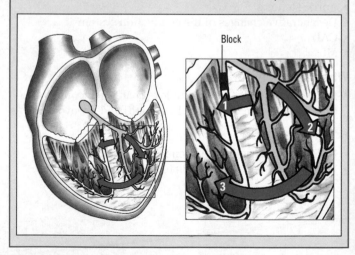

Block

Recognizing RBBB

This 12-lead ECG shows the characteristic changes of RBBB. In lead V_1, note the rsR′ pattern and T-wave inversion. In lead V_6, note the widened S wave and the upright T wave. Also note the prolonged QRS complexes.

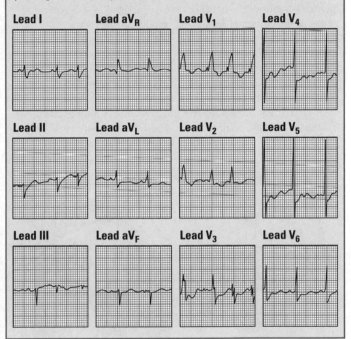

Lead I	Lead aV_R	Lead V_1	Lead V_4
Lead II	Lead aV_L	Lead V_2	Lead V_5
Lead III	Lead aV_F	Lead V_3	Lead V_6

Understanding LBBB

In LBBB, an impulse first travels down the right bundle branch (arrow 1). Then it activates the interventricular septum from right to left (arrow 2) ventricle, the opposite of normal activation. Finally, the impulse activates the left ventricle (arrow 3).

On an ECG, the QRS complex exceeds 0.12 second because the ventricles are activated sequentially, not simultaneously. As the wave of depolarization spreads from the right ventricle to the left, a wide S wave appears in lead V_1 with a positive T wave. The S wave may be preceded by a Q wave or a small R wave.

In lead V_6, no initial Q wave occurs. A tall, notched R wave, or a slurred one, appears as the impulse spreads from right to left. This initial positive deflection is a sign of LBBB. The T wave is negative.

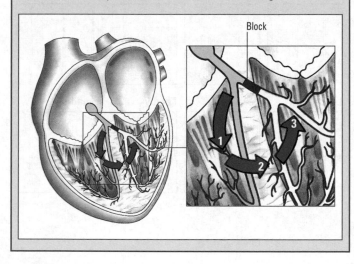

Block

Recognizing LBBB

This 12-lead ECG shows characteristic changes of LBBB. All leads have prolonged QRS complexes. In lead V_1, note the QS wave pattern. In lead V_6, note the slurred R wave and T-wave inversion. The elevated ST segments and upright T waves in leads V_1 to V_4 are also common in this condition.

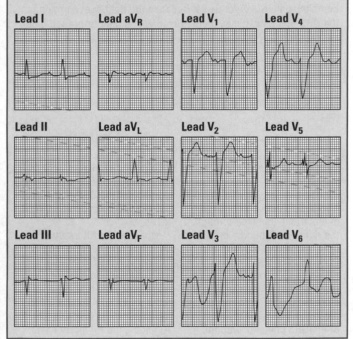

Distinguishing BBB from WPW syndrome

WPW syndrome is a common type of preexcitation syndrome, an abnormal condition in which electrical impulses enter the ventricles from the atria using an accessory pathway that bypasses the AV junction. This results in a short PR interval and a wide QRS complex with an initial slurring of the upward slope of the QRS complex, called a *delta wave*. Because the delta wave prolongs the QRS complex, it may be confused with a bundle-branch block.

BBB

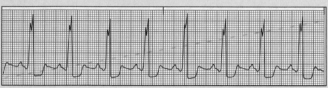

• Carefully examine the QRS complex, noting which part of the complex is widened. A BBB involves defective conduction of electrical impulses through the right or left bundle branch from the bundle of His to the Purkinje network.

• This conduction disturbance results either in an overall increase in QRS duration or a widening of the last part of the QRS complex with the initial part of the QRS complex commonly appearing normal.

• Carefully examine the 12-lead ECG. With a BBB, the prolonged duration of the QRS complexes usually will be consistent in all leads.

• Measure the PR interval. A BBB has no effect on the PR interval, so the PR intervals typically are normal. Keep in mind, however, that if the patient has an AV conduction defect, such as first-degree AV block, the PR interval will be prolonged.

Distinguishing BBB from WPW syndrome *(continued)*

WPW syndrome

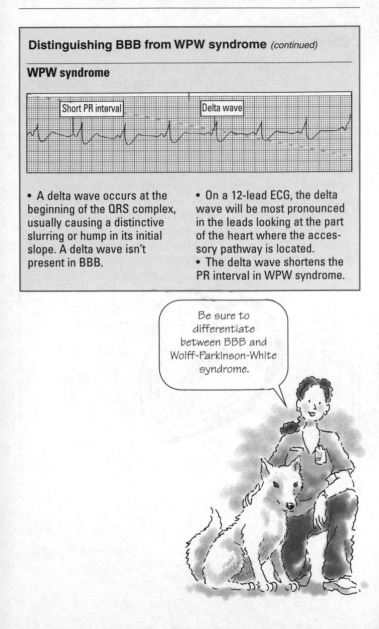

• A delta wave occurs at the beginning of the QRS complex, usually causing a distinctive slurring or hump in its initial slope. A delta wave isn't present in BBB.

• On a 12-lead ECG, the delta wave will be most pronounced in the leads looking at the part of the heart where the accessory pathway is located.
• The delta wave shortens the PR interval in WPW syndrome.

Be sure to differentiate between BBB and Wolff-Parkinson-White syndrome.

Conduction in WPW syndrome

Electrical impulses don't always follow normal conduction pathways in the heart. In preexcitation syndromes, electrical impulses enter the ventricles from the atria through an accessory pathway that bypasses the AV junction. WPW syndrome is a common type of preexcitation syndrome.

WPW syndrome commonly occurs in young children and in adults ages 20 to 35. The syndrome causes the PR interval to shorten and the QRS complex to lengthen as a result of a delta wave. Delta waves, which occur just before normal ventricular depolarization in WPW syndrome, are produced as a result of premature depolarization (preexcitation) of a portion of the ventricles.

WPW syndrome is clinically significant because the accessory pathway—in this case, Kent's bundle—may result in paroxysmal tachyarrhythmias by reentry and rapid conduction mechanisms.

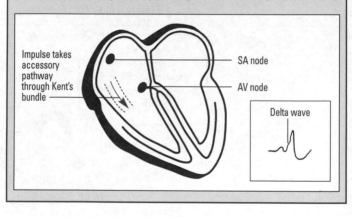

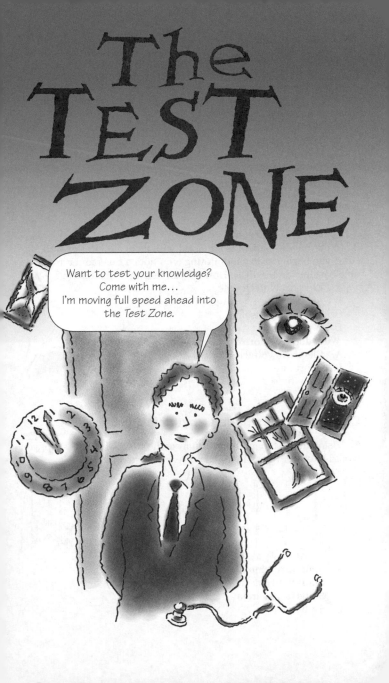

Chapter 1: Basic electrocardiography

1. The six limb leads of a 12-lead ECG provide information about what area of the patient's heart?
   A. Horizontal plane
   B. Frontal plane
   C. Vertical plane
   D. Posterior plane

2. The duration of a normal PR interval is:
   A. 0.04 to 0.08 second.
   B. 0.06 to 0.10 second.
   C. 0.12 to 0.20 second.
   D. 0.24 to 0.36 second.

3. A 60-year-old patient is admitted with an acute inferior wall MI. After you begin cardiac monitoring, you note a thick and unreadable baseline on the ECG. How do you interpret this finding?
   A. Electrical interference
   B. Artifact
   C. Wandering baseline
   D. Weak signal

4. What does the horizontal axis of an ECG represent?
   A. Electrical voltage
   B. Heart rate
   C. Amplitude
   D. Time

Chapter 2: Sinus node arrhythmias

5. Using the 8-step method to analyze the following ECG strip, you would interpret the arrhythmia represented as:

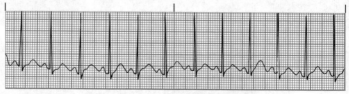

   A. Sinus arrhythmia
   B. Sinus bradycardia
   C. Sinus tachycardia
   D. SA block

6. Which arrhythmia is characterized by a rate that's usually within normal limits but a rhythm that's irregular and corresponds to the respiratory cycle?
   A. Sinus bradycardia
   B. Sinus arrhythmia
   C. Normal sinus rhythm
   D. Sinus arrest

7. ECG characteristics of sick sinus syndrome include:
   A. atrial and ventricular rates interrupted by a long sinus pause.
   B. regular atrial and ventricular rhythms.
   C. consistently prolonged PR intervals.
   D. wide and bizarre QRS complexes.

Chapter 3: Atrial arrhythmias

8. The characteristic features of a PAC include:
   A. P waves replaced by waveforms with a sawtooth appearance.
   B. P wave followed by a wide, bizarre QRS complex.
   C. inverted P waves.
   D. premature, abnormally-shaped P waves.

9. You notice the following rhythm on a patient's monitor and obtain a rhythm strip. After examining the characteristics of the strip, you identify the rhythm as:

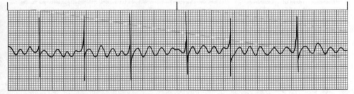

   A. atrial flutter.
   B. atrial fibrillation.
   C. normal sinus rhythm with PACs.
   D. wandering pacemaker.

10. Carotid massage may be used to:
   A. suppress the ectopic focus of PACs.
   B. convert PAT to normal sinus rhythm.
   C. suppress the chaotic atrial activity in atrial fibrillation.
   D. convert wandering pacemaker to normal sinus rhythm.

Chapter 4: Junctional arrhythmias

11. In a PJC, the P wave can occur:
A. upright before the QRS complex.
B. within the ST segment.
C. inverted before, during, or after the QRS complex.
D. within the T wave.

12. In junctional rhythm, you would expect the rate to be between:
A. 20 and 40 beats/minute.
B. 40 and 60 beats/minute.
C. 60 and 80 beats/minute.
D. 80 and 100 beats/minute.

13. In junctional tachycardia, the PR interval is generally:
A. shortened and less than 0.12 second.
B. shortened and less than 0.04 second.
C. prolonged and greater than 0.20 second.
D. not measurable because P waves are absent.

14. Characteristics of a junctional rhythm include:
A. regular rhythm and a wide QRS complex.
B. regular rhythm and a narrow QRS complex.
C. irregular rhythm and a wide QRS complex.
D. irregular rhythm and the presence of U waves.

Chapter 5: Ventricular arrhythmias

15. A patient is admitted with an acute MI and suddenly develops the rhythm shown below. The treatment of choice for this rhythm is:

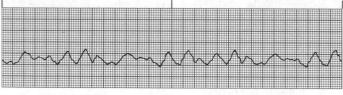

A. synchronized cardioversion.
B. atropine.
C. defibrillation.
D. transesophageal pacing.

16. Treatment of idioventricular rhythm typically includes:
  A. amiodarone.
  B. transcutaneous pacing.
  C. lidocaine.
  D. synchronized cardioversion.

17. A patient with a low magnesium level develops an arrhythmia. You record the rhythm strip below and identify the arrhythmia as:
  A. supraventricular tachycardia.
  B. ventricular fibrillation.
  C. ventricular flutter.
  D. torsades de pointes.

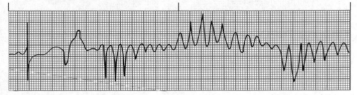

Chapter 6: Atrioventricular blocks

18. First-degree AV block is characterized by a PR interval that exceeds:
  A. 0.16 second.
  B. 0.20 second.
  C. 0.24 second.
  D. 0.32 second.

19. In type I second-degree AV block, the PR interval:
  A. isn't measurable.
  B. remains constant.
  C. varies according to the ventricular rate.
  D. progressively lengthens until a P wave appears without a QRS complex.

20. You would identify the rhythm in the strip shown below as:
   A. first-degree AV block.
   B. type II second-degree AV block.
   C. third-degree AV block.
   D. type I second-degree AV block.

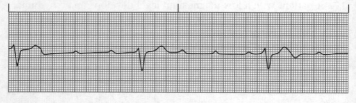

Chapter 7: ECG effects of electrolyte imbalances

21. Which electrolyte imbalance commonly causes classic tall, peaked T waves on an ECG?
   A. Hyperkalemia
   B. Hypokalemia
   C. Hypercalcemia
   D. Hypocalcemia

22. Which electrolyte imbalance commonly causes a flattened T wave and the appearance of a U wave on an ECG?
   A. Hyperkalemia
   B. Hypokalemia
   C. Hypercalcemia
   D. Hypocalcemia

23. Which ECG finding would be seen on the ECG of the patient with hypocalcemia?
   A. Prolonged PR interval
   B. Peaked T waves
   C. Shortened QT interval
   D. Prolonged QT interval

24. Causes of hyperkalemia may include:
   A. burns, massive crush injuries, and Addison's disease.
   B. diarrhea, intestinal fistulae, and vomiting.
   C. bone metastasis, sarcoidosis, and hyperparathyroidism.
   D. pancreatitis, excessive phosphorus intake, and vomiting.

Chapter 8: ECG effects of antiarrhythmics

25. The following ECG strip shows the characteristic effect of which of the following cardiac drugs?

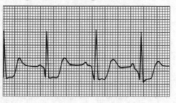

    A. Mexiletine
    B. Procainamide
    C. Digoxin
    D. Sotalol

26. Class IA antiarrhythmic drugs may produce which ECG effect?
    A. Prolonged QT interval and slightly widened QRS complex
    B. Shortened QT interval and slightly widened QRS complex
    C. Prolonged PR interval and peaked T wave
    D. Shortened PR interval and shortened QT interval

27. Class III antiarrhythmic drugs increase the duration of the action potential and block potassium during phase 3 of the action potential. Which of the following drugs is classified as a class III antiarrhythmic?
    A. Disopyramide
    B. Ibutilide
    C. Tocainide
    D. Esmolol

Chapter 9: Pacemakers and ICDs

28. You're caring for a patient who developed complications after an acute MI requiring a transvenous pacemaker insertion. His monitor alarm sounds and the rhythm strip shown below is recorded. You interpret this rhythm as which type of pacemaker malfunction?

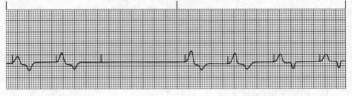

- A. Failure to capture
- B. Failure to pace
- C. Failure to sense (undersensing)
- D. Oversensing

29. When teaching a patient with a newly inserted permanent pacemaker, you should:

- A. advise him that exposure to strong electromagnetic fields is safe.
- B. tell him that hiccups are normal for the first few days after pacemaker insertion.
- C. instruct him to avoid tight clothing.
- D. explain that MRI scans are safe.

30. An ICD may be programmed to detect which of the following arrhythmias?

- A. Ventricular tachycardia, ventricular fibrillation, junctional tachycardia, and asystole
- B. Ventricular fibrillation only
- C. Ventricular tachycardia and ventricular fibrillation only
- D. Ventricular tachycardia, ventricular fibrillation, bradycardia, and atrial fibrillation

Chapter 10: Basic 12-lead electrocardiography

31. Leads II, III, and aV$_F$ look at which area of the heart?

- A. Inferior wall
- B. Lateral wall
- C. Anterior wall
- D. Septal wall

32. Which lead placement is the correct one for precordial lead V_2?
   A.   Fourth intercostal space, right sternal border
   B.   Fourth intercostal space, left sternal border
   C.   Fifth intercostal space, left midclavicular line
   D.   Fifth intercostal space, left midaxillary line

33. A 12-lead ECG is used to assess function of the:
   A.   left atrium.
   B.   right and left ventricles simultaneously.
   C.   left ventricle.
   D.   right ventricle.

34. Right precordial leads can provide specific information about the functioning of the:
   A.   left ventricle.
   B.   right ventricle.
   C.   left atrium.
   D.   right atrium.

Chapter 11: Advanced electrocardiography

35. Myocardial injury is represented on an ECG by the presence of:
   A.   prolonged QT interval and T-wave inversion.
   B.   ST-segment elevation and pathologic Q waves.
   C.   ST-segment elevation and T-wave inversion.
   D.   T-wave inversion and pathologic Q waves.

36. Your patient's ECG shows a QRS complex with a positive deflection in lead I and a negative deflection in lead aV_F. Using the four-quadrant method for determining electrical axis, you determine he has:
   A.   right axis deviation.
   B.   left axis deviation.
   C.   normal axis.
   D.   extreme right axis deviation.

37. When examining your patient's 12-lead ECG, you notice a bundle-branch block. Which leads should you check to determine whether the block is in the right or left bundle?
   A. V_1 and V_6
   B. V_4 and V_5
   C.   II and aV_L
   D.   I and V_6

38. A 52-year-old patient is admitted after a recent bacterial respiratory infection. He complains of chest pain that increases on deep inspiration. His 12-lead ECG shows diffuse ST-segment elevation in most limb and precordial leads. The most likely diagnosis is:

    A. acute inferior-wall MI.

    B. acute anterior-wall MI.

    C. Prinzmetal's angina.

    D. acute pericarditis.

Answers

Chapter 1: Basic electrocardiography

1. B. The six limb leads: leads I, II, III, aV_R, aV_L, and aV_F, provide information about the heart's frontal plane.
2. C. The duration of a normal PR interval is 0.12 to 0.20 second.
3. A. Electrical interference appears on the ECG as a baseline that's thick and unreadable. Also called *AC interference*, it's caused by electrical power leakage or improperly grounded equipment in the room.
4. D. The horizontal axis of an ECG strip represents time.

Chapter 2: Sinus node arrhythmias

5. C. Interpretation: Sinus tachycardia
Rhythm: Regular atrial and ventricular rhythms
Rate: Atrial and ventricular 115 beats/minute
P wave: Normal size and configuration
PR interval: 0.14 second
QRS complex: 0.06 second, normal size and configuration
T wave: Normal size and configuration
QT interval: 0.34 second
6. B. In sinus arrhythmia, the rate is usually within normal limits, but the rhythm is irregular and corresponds to the respiratory cycle. Sinus arrhythmia may occur with bradycardia and is referred to as a *sinus bradyarrhythmia*.
7. A. Sick sinus syndrome is characterized by atrial and ventricular rates that are slow, fast, or alternate between slow and fast and are interrupted by a long sinus pause.

Chapter 3: Atrial arrhythmias

8. D. Because PACs originate in the atria rather than in the SA node, the P wave has a different configuration than the sinus P wave and occurs early in the cardiac cycle.
9. A. Atrial flutter with flutter waves replacing the P waves has a baseline with a characteristic sawtooth appearance.

10. B. Carotid massage stimulates the vagus nerve, which then inhibits firing of the SA node and slows AV conduction. This allows the SA node to reset itself as the primary pacemaker.

Chapter 4: Junctional arrhythmias

11. C. In a PJC, the P wave is inverted (leads II, III, and aV_F) and may occur before, during, or after the QRS complex. If the atria and ventricles depolarize simultaneously, the P wave is hidden in the QRS complex.

12. B. In junctional rhythm, the rate is between 40 and 60 beats/minute. This is the inherent rate of the AV junction.

13. A. If the P wave precedes the QRS complex, the PR interval is measurable and is less than 0.12 second.

14. B. Junctional rhythm is characterized by a regular rhythm and a QRS complex duration within normal limits.

Chapter 5: Ventricular arrhythmias

15. C. A patient in ventricular fibrillation is in cardiac arrest and requires immediate defibrillation.

16. B. Transcutaneous pacing is a temporary way to increase the patient's heart rate and ensure adequate cardiac output, particularly in patients who don't respond to atropine. This rhythm is never treated with antiarrhythmic drugs that would suppress the escape beats because it could lead to ventricular standstill.

17. D. This rhythm strip shows torsades de pointes with characteristic phasic variation in electrical polarity, with wide QRS complexes that point downward for several beats and then upward for several beats.

Chapter 6: Atrioventricular blocks

18. B. First-degree AV block is characterized by a PR interval that exceeds 0.20 second.

19. D. In type I second-degree AV block, progressive lengthening of the PR interval occurs until a P wave appears without a QRS complex.

20. C. This strip shows third-degree AV block. Because the atria and ventricles beat independently of each other in third-degree AV block, the PR interval varies with each beat and, therefore, isn't measurable.

Chapter 7: ECG effects of electrolyte imbalances

21. A. The presence of tall, peaked T waves is characteristic of hyperkalemia.

22. B. The presence of a U wave and a flattened T wave are characteristic of hypokalemia.

23. D. Prolonged QT interval is the key finding on the ECG of a patient with hypocalcemia.

24. A. Conditions that may cause hyperkalemia include burns, massive crush injuries, and Addison's disease as well as renal failure and use of potassium-sparing diuretics.

Chapter 8: ECG effects of antiarrhythmics

25. C. Digoxin, a cardiac glycoside, typically causes a characteristic sagging of the ST segment.

26. A. Class IA antiarrhythmic drugs may slightly widen the QRS complex and prolong the QT interval. Increased widening of the QRS complex is an early sign of toxicity, and the prolonged QT interval predisposes the patient to polymorphic ventricular tachycardia.

27. B. Ibutilide is a class III antiarrhythmic that's used for rapid conversion of recent-onset atrial fibrillation or atrial flutter.

Chapter 9: Pacemakers and ICDs

28. A. The rhythm strip shows the pacemaker's failure to capture. The ECG pacemaker spike isn't followed by a QRS complex.

29. C. You should instruct the patient to avoid tight clothing or direct pressure over the pulse generator, avoid exposure to strong electromagnetic fields, avoid MRI scans and certain other diagnostic studies, and notify the doctor if he feels confused, light-headed, or short of breath or has palpitations, hiccups, or a rapid or unusually slow pulse rate.

30. D. An ICD may be programmed to detect ventricular tachycardia, ventricular fibrillation, bradycardia, and atrial fibrillation.

Chapter 10: Basic 12-lead electrocardiography

31. A. Leads II, III, and aV_F look at the inferior wall of the heart.

32. B. Lead V_2 is placed over the fourth intercostal space at the left sternal border.

33. C. A 12-lead ECG gives a more complete review of the heart's electrical activity than a rhythm strip and is used to assess left ventricular function.

34. B. Right precordial leads provide specific information about the function of the right ventricle.

Chapter 11: Advanced electrocardiography

35. C. ST-segment elevation and T-wave inversion are the ECG changes that correspond with myocardial injury.

36. B. When lead I points upward and lead aV_F points downward, left axis deviation exists.

37. A. After you identify a bundle-branch block, examine lead V_1, which lies to the right of the heart, and lead V_6, which lies to the left of the heart. These leads tell you if the block is in the right or left bundle branch.

38. D. Pericarditis is commonly caused by a recent infection and is characterized by chest pain that increases on deep inspiration. ECG changes include diffuse ST-segment elevations, typically in leads I, II, III, aV_L, aV_F, and V_2 through V_6.

Scoring

☆☆☆ If you answered 35 to 38 questions correctly, great job! You're in a dimension all by yourself.

☆☆ If you answered 30 to 34 questions correctly, way to go! You're really in the zone.

☆ If you answered fewer than 30 questions correctly, review the chapters and try again! It won't be long until you see the light.

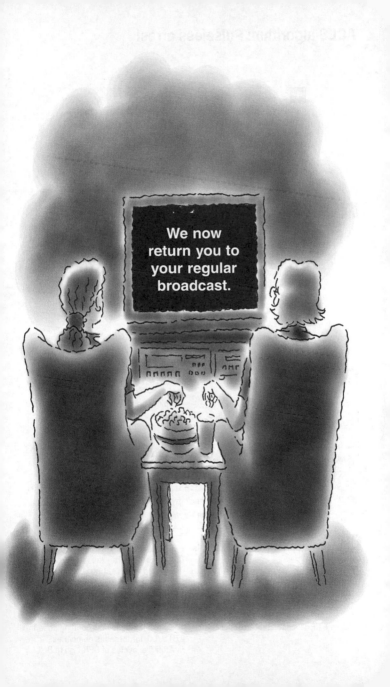

ACLS algorithm: Pulseless arrest

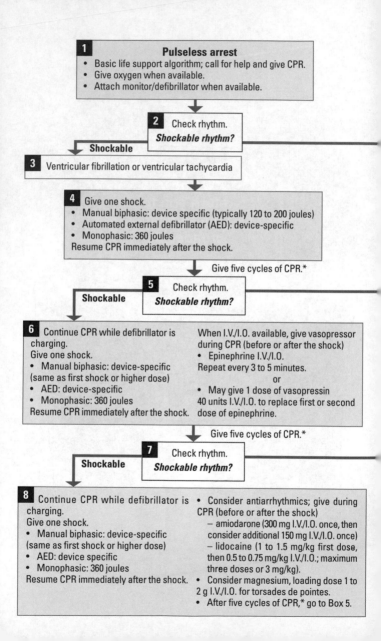

1 Pulseless arrest
- Basic life support algorithm; call for help and give CPR.
- Give oxygen when available.
- Attach monitor/defibrillator when available.

2 Check rhythm.
Shockable rhythm?

Shockable

3 Ventricular fibrillation or ventricular tachycardia

4 Give one shock.
- Manual biphasic: device specific (typically 120 to 200 joules)
- Automated external defibrillator (AED): device-specific
- Monophasic: 360 joules
Resume CPR immediately after the shock.

Give five cycles of CPR.*

5 Check rhythm.
Shockable rhythm?

Shockable

6 Continue CPR while defibrillator is charging.
Give one shock.
- Manual biphasic: device-specific (same as first shock or higher dose)
- AED: device-specific
- Monophasic: 360 joules
Resume CPR immediately after the shock.

When I.V./I.O. available, give vasopressor during CPR (before or after the shock)
- Epinephrine I.V./I.O.
Repeat every 3 to 5 minutes.
or
- May give 1 dose of vasopressin 40 units I.V./I.O. to replace first or second dose of epinephrine.

Give five cycles of CPR.*

7 Check rhythm.
Shockable rhythm?

Shockable

8 Continue CPR while defibrillator is charging.
Give one shock.
- Manual biphasic: device-specific (same as first shock or higher dose)
- AED: device specific
- Monophasic: 360 joules
Resume CPR immediately after the shock.

- Consider antiarrhythmics; give during CPR (before or after the shock)
  – amiodarone (300 mg I.V./I.O. once, then consider additional 150 mg I.V./I.O. once)
  – lidocaine (1 to 1.5 mg/kg first dose, then 0.5 to 0.75 mg/kg I.V./I.O.; maximum three doses or 3 mg/kg).
- Consider magnesium, loading dose 1 to 2 g I.V./I.O. for torsades de pointes.
- After five cycles of CPR,* go to Box 5.

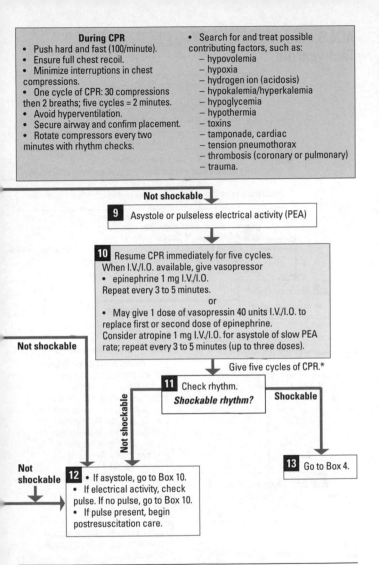

During CPR
- Push hard and fast (100/minute).
- Ensure full chest recoil.
- Minimize interruptions in chest compressions.
- One cycle of CPR: 30 compressions then 2 breaths; five cycles = 2 minutes.
- Avoid hyperventilation.
- Secure airway and confirm placement.
- Rotate compressors every two minutes with rhythm checks.

- Search for and treat possible contributing factors, such as:
  – hypovolemia
  – hypoxia
  – hydrogen ion (acidosis)
  – hypokalemia/hyperkalemia
  – hypoglycemia
  – hypothermia
  – toxins
  – tamponade, cardiac
  – tension pneumothorax
  – thrombosis (coronary or pulmonary)
  – trauma.

Not shockable

9 Asystole or pulseless electrical activity (PEA)

10 Resume CPR immediately for five cycles.
When I.V./I.O. available, give vasopressor
- epinephrine 1 mg I.V./I.O.
Repeat every 3 to 5 minutes.

or

- May give 1 dose of vasopressin 40 units I.V./I.O. to replace first or second dose of epinephrine.
Consider atropine 1 mg I.V./I.O. for asystole of slow PEA rate; repeat every 3 to 5 minutes (up to three doses).

Give five cycles of CPR.*

11 Check rhythm.
Shockable rhythm?

Not shockable

Shockable

Not shockable

13 Go to Box 4.

Not shockable

12
- If asystole, go to Box 10.
- If electrical activity, check pulse. If no pulse, go to Box 10.
- If pulse present, begin postresuscitation care.

* After an advanced airway is placed, rescuers no longer deliver "cycles" of CPR. Give continuous chest compressions without pauses for breaths. Give 8 to 10 breaths/minute. Check rhythm every 2 minutes.

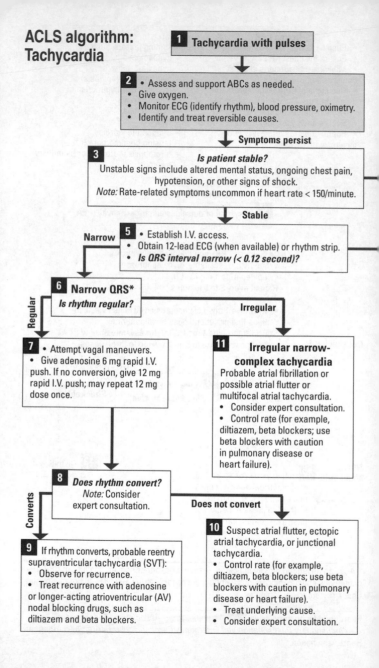

ACLS algorithm: Tachycardia

1 **Tachycardia with pulses**

2
- Assess and support ABCs as needed.
- Give oxygen.
- Monitor ECG (identify rhythm), blood pressure, oximetry.
- Identify and treat reversible causes.

Symptoms persist

3
Is patient stable?
Unstable signs include altered mental status, ongoing chest pain, hypotension, or other signs of shock.
Note: Rate-related symptoms uncommon if heart rate < 150/minute.

Stable

5 **Narrow**
- Establish I.V. access.
- Obtain 12-lead ECG (when available) or rhythm strip.
- *Is QRS interval narrow (< 0.12 second)?*

6 **Narrow QRS***
Is rhythm regular?

Regular

Irregular

7
- Attempt vagal maneuvers.
- Give adenosine 6 mg rapid I.V. push. If no conversion, give 12 mg rapid I.V. push; may repeat 12 mg dose once.

11
Irregular narrow-complex tachycardia
Probable atrial fibrillation or possible atrial flutter or multifocal atrial tachycardia.
- Consider expert consultation.
- Control rate (for example, diltiazem, beta blockers; use beta blockers with caution in pulmonary disease or heart failure).

8
Does rhythm convert?
Note: Consider expert consultation.

Converts

Does not convert

9 If rhythm converts, probable reentry supraventricular tachycardia (SVT):
- Observe for recurrence.
- Treat recurrence with adenosine or longer-acting atrioventricular (AV) nodal blocking drugs, such as diltiazem and beta blockers.

10 Suspect atrial flutter, ectopic atrial tachycardia, or junctional tachycardia.
- Control rate (for example, diltiazem, beta blockers; use beta blockers with caution in pulmonary disease or heart failure).
- Treat underlying cause.
- Consider expert consultation.

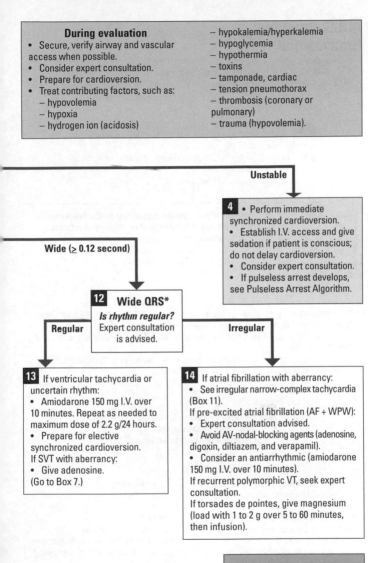

During evaluation
- Secure, verify airway and vascular access when possible.
- Consider expert consultation.
- Prepare for cardioversion.
- Treat contributing factors, such as:
  – hypovolemia
  – hypoxia
  – hydrogen ion (acidosis)
  – hypokalemia/hyperkalemia
  – hypoglycemia
  – hypothermia
  – toxins
  – tamponade, cardiac
  – tension pneumothorax
  – thrombosis (coronary or pulmonary)
  – trauma (hypovolemia).

Unstable

4
- Perform immediate synchronized cardioversion.
- Establish I.V. access and give sedation if patient is conscious; do not delay cardioversion.
- Consider expert consultation.
- If pulseless arrest develops, see Pulseless Arrest Algorithm.

Wide (≥ 0.12 second)

12   Wide QRS*
Is rhythm regular?
Expert consultation is advised.

Regular

Irregular

13 If ventricular tachycardia or uncertain rhythm:
- Amiodarone 150 mg I.V. over 10 minutes. Repeat as needed to maximum dose of 2.2 g/24 hours.
- Prepare for elective synchronized cardioversion.
If SVT with aberrancy:
- Give adenosine.
(Go to Box 7.)

14 If atrial fibrillation with aberrancy:
- See irregular narrow-complex tachycardia (Box 11).
If pre-excited atrial fibrillation (AF + WPW):
- Expert consultation advised.
- Avoid AV-nodal-blocking agents (adenosine, digoxin, diltiazem, and verapamil).
- Consider an antiarrhythmic (amiodarone 150 mg I.V. over 10 minutes).
If recurrent polymorphic VT, seek expert consultation.
If torsades de pointes, give magnesium (load with 1 to 2 g over 5 to 60 minutes, then infusion).

***Note: If patient becomes unstable, go to Box 4.**

Reproduced with permission, *2005 American Heart Association Guidelines for Cardiopulmonary Resuscitation and Emergency Cardiovascular Care* © 2005 American Heart Association.

ACLS algorithm: Bradycardia

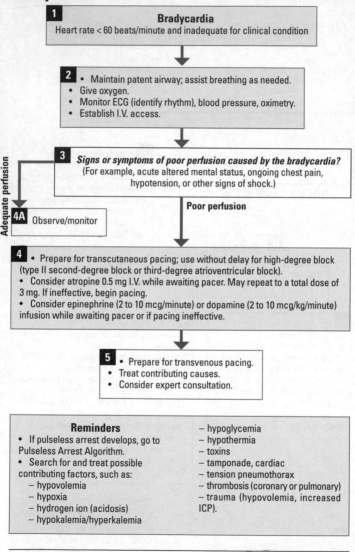

1

Bradycardia
Heart rate < 60 beats/minute and inadequate for clinical condition

2
- Maintain patent airway; assist breathing as needed.
- Give oxygen.
- Monitor ECG (identify rhythm), blood pressure, oximetry.
- Establish I.V. access.

3
Signs or symptoms of poor perfusion caused by the bradycardia?
(For example, acute altered mental status, ongoing chest pain, hypotension, or other signs of shock.)

Adequate perfusion

Poor perfusion

4A Observe/monitor

4
- Prepare for transcutaneous pacing; use without delay for high-degree block (type II second-degree block or third-degree atrioventricular block).
- Consider atropine 0.5 mg I.V. while awaiting pacer. May repeat to a total dose of 3 mg. If ineffective, begin pacing.
- Consider epinephrine (2 to 10 mcg/minute) or dopamine (2 to 10 mcg/kg/minute) infusion while awaiting pacer or if pacing ineffective.

5
- Prepare for transvenous pacing.
- Treat contributing causes.
- Consider expert consultation.

Reminders
- If pulseless arrest develops, go to Pulseless Arrest Algorithm.
- Search for and treat possible contributing factors, such as:
  – hypovolemia
  – hypoxia
  – hydrogen ion (acidosis)
  – hypokalemia/hyperkalemia
  – hypoglycemia
  – hypothermia
  – toxins
  – tamponade, cardiac
  – tension pneumothorax
  – thrombosis (coronary or pulmonary)
  – trauma (hypovolemia, increased ICP).

Guide to antiarrhythmic drugs

This chart details the drugs most commonly used to manage cardiac arrhythmias, including indications and special considerations for each.

Drugs	Indications	Special considerations
Class IA antiarrhythmics Disopyramide, procainamide, quinidine	• Ventricular tachycardia (VT) • Atrial fibrillation • Atrial flutter • Paroxysmal atrial tachycardia (PAT)	• Check apical pulse rate before therapy. If you note extremes in pulse rate, withhold the dose and notify the prescriber. • Use cautiously in patients with reactive airway disease, such as asthma. • Monitor for ECG changes (widening QRS complexes, prolonged QT interval).
Class IB antiarrhythmics Lidocaine, mexiletine	• VT • Ventricular fibrillation (VF)	• IB antiarrhythmics may potentiate the effects of other antiarrhythmics. • Administer I.V. infusions using an infusion pump.
Class IC antiarrhythmics Flecainide, propafenone	• VT • VF • Supraventricular arrhythmias	• Correct electrolyte imbalances before administration. • Monitor the patient's ECG before and after dosage adjustments. • Monitor hepatic and renal function for toxicity.

Drugs	Indications	Special considerations
Class II antiarrhythmics Acebutolol, atenolol, propranolol	• Atrial flutter • Atrial fibrillation • PAT	• Monitor apical heart rate and blood pressure. • Abruptly stopping these drugs can exacerbate angina and precipitate myocardial infarction. • Monitor for ECG changes (prolonged PR interval). • Drugs may mask common signs and symptoms of shock and hypoglycemia. • Use with caution in patients with reactive airway disease, such as asthma.
Class III antiarrhythmics Amiodarone	• Life-threatening arrhythmias resistant to other antiarrhythmic drugs	• Monitor blood pressure and heart rate and rhythm for changes. • Amiodarone increases the risk of digoxin toxicity in patients also taking digoxin. • Monitor for signs of pulmonary toxicity (crackles, dyspnea, and pleuritic chest pain), thyroid dysfunction, and vision impairment in patients taking amiodarone. • Monitor for ECG changes (prolonged QT interval) in patients taking dofetilide, ibutilide, and sotalol.

Drugs	Indications	Special considerations
Class IV antiarrhythmics		
Diltiazem, verapamil	• Supraventricular arrhythmias	• Monitor heart rate and rhythm and blood pressure carefully when initiating therapy or increasing dose. • Calcium supplements may reduce effectiveness.
Miscellaneous antiarrhythmics		
Adenosine	• Paroxysmal supraventricular tachycardia	• Adenosine must be administered over 1 to 2 seconds, followed by a 20-ml flush of normal saline solution. • Record rhythm strip during administration. Adenosine may cause transient asystole or heart block.
Atropine	• Symptomatic sinus bradycardia • AV block • Asystole • Bradycardic pulseless electrical activity (PEA)	• Monitor cardiac rate and rhythm. Use the drug cautiously in patients with myocardial ischemia. • Atropine isn't recommended for third-degree AV block or infranodal type II second-degree AV block. • In adults, avoid doses less than 0.5 mg because the risk of paradoxical slowing of the heart rate.

Drugs	Indications	Special considerations
Miscellaneous antiarrhythmics *(continued)*		
Epinephrine	• Pulseless VT • VF • Asystole • PEA	• Monitor cardiac rate and rhythm and blood pressure carefully because the drug may cause myocardial ischemia. • Don't mix an I.V. dose with alkaline solutions. • Give drug into a large vein to prevent irritation or extravasation at site.
Vasopressin	• VF that's unresponsive to defibrillation	• Monitor cardiac rate and rhythm. Use the drug cautiously in patients with myocardial ischemia. • Monitor for hypersensitivity reactions, especially urticaria, angioedema, and bronchoconstriction.

Choosing monitoring leads

Most bedside monitoring systems allow for simultaneous monitoring of two leads, such as lead II with V_1 or MCL_1. Lead II or the lead that clearly shows the P waves and QRS complex may be used for sinus node arrhythmias, premature atrial contractions, and atrioventricular block. The precordial leads V_1 and V_6 or the bipolar leads MCL_1 and MCL_6 are the best leads for monitoring rhythms with wide QRS complexes and for differentiating ventricular tachycardia from supraventricular tachycardia with aberrancy.

The table below lists the best leads for monitoring challenging cardiac arrhythmias.

Arrhythmia	Best monitoring leads
• Premature atrial contractions	II or lead that shows best P waves
• Atrial tachycardia	II, V_1, V_6, MCL_1, MCL_6
• Paroxysmal atrial tachycardia	II, V_1, V_6, MCL_1, MCL_6
• Atrial flutter	II, III
• Atrial fibrillation	II (or identified in most leads by fibrillatory waves and irregular R-R)
• Premature junctional contractions	II
• Junctional escape rhythm	II
• Junctional tachycardia	II, V_1, V_6, MCL_1, MCL_6
• Premature ventricular contractions	V_1, V_6, MCL_1, MCL_6
• Idioventricular rhythm	V_1, V_6, MCL_1, MCL_6
• Ventricular tachycardia	V_1, V_6, MCL_1, MCL_6
• Ventricular fibrillation	Any
• Torsades de pointes	Any
• Third-degree AV block	II or lead that shows best P waves and QRS complexes

Selected references

"AHA Scientific Statement: Practice Standards for Electrocardiographic Monitoring in Hospital Setting," *Circulation* 110:2721–46, 2004.

American College of Cardiology and American Heart Association. "ACC/AHA Clinical Competence Statement on Electrocardiography and Ambulatory Electrocardiography," *Circulation* 104(25):3169–78, December 2001.

"2005 American Heart Association Guidelines for Cardiopulmonary Resuscitation and Emergency Cardiovascular Care," *Circulation* 112(suppl. IV): IV-58-IV-66, 2005.

Brantman, L., and Howie, J. "Use of Amiodarone to Prevent Atrial Fibrillation after Cardiac Surgery," *Critical Care Nurse* 26(1):48–56, 58; quiz 59, February 2006.

Cardiovascular Care Made Incredibly Easy. Philadelphia, Pa.: Lippincott Williams & Wilkins, 2005.

Coady, E. "Managing Patients with Non-ST-Segment Elevation Acute Coronary Syndrome," *Nursing Standard* 20(37):49–56, May 2006.

Cuisset, T., et al. "Benefit of a 600-mg Loading Dose of Clopidogrel on Platelet Reactivity and Clinical Outcomes in Patients with Non-ST-Segment Elevation Acute Coronary Syndrome Undergoing Coronary Stenting," *Journal of the American College of Cardiology* 48(7): 1339–45, October 2006.

Davies, A. "Recognizing and Reducing Interference on 12-lead Electrocardiograms," *British Journal of Nursing* 16(13):800–4, July 2007.

Fugate, J.H. "Pharmacologic Management of Cardiac Emergencies," *Journal of Infusion Nursing* 29(3): 147–50, May–June 2006.

Jones, S. *ECG Notes: Interpretation and Management Guide.* Philadelphia: F.A. Davis Co., 2005.

Jowett, N.I., et al. "Modified Electrode Placement

Must Be Recorded When Performing 12-lead Electrocardiograms," *Postgraduate Medical Journal* 81(952):122–25, February 2005.

Lim, W., et al. "Reliability of Electrocardiogram Interpretation in Critically Ill Patients," *Critical Care Medicine* 34(5):1338–43, May 2006.

Pyne, C. "Classification of Acute Coronary Syndromes Using the 12-Lead Electro-cardiogram as a Guide," *AACN Clinical Issues: Advanced Practice* 15(4): October/December 2004.

Tsiperfal, A. "What is Drug-induced Long QT and What Is a Potential Clinical Consequence?" *Progress in Cardio-vascular Nursing* 21(2):104–5, Spring 2006.

Wysocki, L. "ST Segment Changes Clue You into Injury Location," *RN* 69(9):49, September 2006.

Index

i refers to an illustration; t refers to a table.

i refers to an illustration; t refers to a table.

i refers to an illustration; t refers to a table.

i refers to an illustration; t refers to a table.